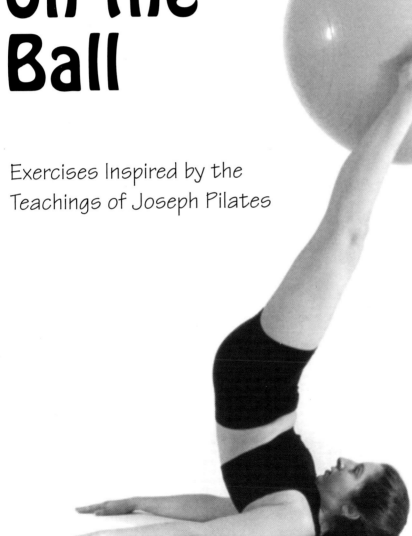

Balance on the Ball

Exercises Inspired by the
Teachings of Joseph Pilates

Balance on the Ball

Exercises Inspired by the Teachings of Joseph Pilates

Elisabeth Crawford

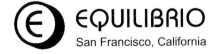

EQUILIBRIO
San Francisco, California

Library of Congress Catalog Card Number: 00-192966
ISBN 0-9703716-0-8

Photography by Steve Savage
Illustrations by Michael Antoine
Design/Layout by Falcon Books

Find us on the World Wide Web at
www.balanceontheball.com

Distributed by:
Equipment Shop
P.O. Box 33
Bedford, MA 01730
1-800-525-7681
www.equipmentshop.com

Notice to Readers: Before following any advice contained in this book, it is recommended that you consult your doctor if you suffer from any health problems or special conditions or are in doubt as to its suitability.

Acknowledgments

The author would like to thank the following people:

Ken Larson of Equipment Shop and Steno Dondè of Ledragomma for their assistance with the production, promotion, and distribution of this book. Their companies provide a valuable service to people in the health and fitness industry worldwide, and I feel honored to be working with both of them.

Steve Savage for his outstanding photography.

Michael Antoine for providing the illustrations and for his never-ending patience.

Joe Ravicini, Alexander Agopovich, and Anda Abramovici for their valuable support and advice.

To all of my students for their dedication and enthusiasm.

A very special thank you to Judy Hummell and Michael Antoine for their unconditional love and support.

ℰ ℛ

Dedicated to my father, James M. Crawford.

Table of Contents

Introduction

Maintaining a balanced, healthy lifestyle has become a predominant value in today's society. The 1990s brought an increased interest in many health-related areas, including nutrition, holistic medicine, and fitness. We are more concerned than ever with taking preventative measures against disease, injury, obesity, and the effects of aging.

There has been a similar shift in the focus of the fitness industry toward prevention, through strengthening the core of the body and understanding proper alignment. We have steered away from the "no pain, no gain" mentality of previous decades and are searching for safer, more gentle ways to stay fit. We are no longer as obsessed with our physical appearance and are becoming more aware of the overall well-being of our bodies. This change in focus explains the recent surge in popularity of both the Ball and the Pilates® method.

The exercises designed by Joseph Pilates strive to create a balanced body, a harmonious structure which performs with efficiency and precision, integrating body and mind. This book draws from his teachings to provide a fun and challenging workout on the Ball for people at all levels of fitness.

History of the Ball

Originally manufactured in Italy, the Ball was first used as a tool for rehabilitation in Switzerland in the 1960s. Dr. Susanne Klein-Vogelbach is believed to be the first physiotherapist to incorporate the Ball in the treatment of patients with orthopedic and neurological disorders. In the 1970s, therapists in the U.S. began using the Ball to treat spinal injuries and other medical problems, but it was not discovered as an effective method of general body conditioning until the early 1990s. The Ball is now widely recognized in the fitness industry, and many personal trainers believe it to be their best overall training tool for developing core strength, flexibility, balance, and posture.

History of the Pilates® Method

Pilates® is a method of exercise and body conditioning that has been practiced since the early 1920s. It was developed by German-born Joseph Pilates who, while working as a nurse in England during World War I, experimented with attaching a system of springs to the hospital beds as a way for patients to begin rehabilitation while still bedridden. This new concept produced dramatic results. Combining his experience as a diver, boxer and gymnast with his studies of yoga, Zen and other Eastern techniques, he eventually evolved this practice into his unique method of physical and mental conditioning.

In 1926 Joseph Pilates emigrated to New York where he began teaching his method to members of the dance world, including the companies of George Balanchine and Martha Graham. His method became the conditioning and rehabilitation method of choice for the dance community and remains so today, due in large part to its emphasis on balance and its treatment of the body as a whole. Until fairly recently, the method has been used almost exclusively by dancers and other artists, but with the recent explosion of media attention, it is becoming more accessible to the general public. The Pilates® exercises are practiced by all types of individuals, from football players to white-collar professionals to Hollywood celebrities. Movements range from basic and rehabilitating for those injured or out of shape to advanced and extremely challenging for the peak-condition athlete.

Benefits of Exercising on the Ball

1. Increases *muscle strength*. This includes muscle tone and definition as well as endurance. Your body weight will provide the resistance in most exercises as you work against gravity, although there are a few exercises where the Ball itself supplies the resistance.

2. Increases *flexibility*, perhaps to a greater degree than performing similar stretches on a stable surface. The Ball allows you to find subtle nuances in every stretch, because by rolling it back and forth, you may stretch different fibers of the same muscle. In addition, many exercises combine both stretching and strengthening of the same muscle, which has been proven to be more effective than plain static stretching.

3. Improves *balance and coordination* on a neuromuscular level. The Ball is a unique exercise tool in that it is not a stable surface. To perform any strengthening or stretching exercise, you must not only use the muscles required to execute the movement, but another set of stabilizing muscles in your torso just to maintain balance. Because balancing on the Ball is a reflex response, it can help you to bypass habitual patterns that interfere with normal functioning. For example, if your body tends to lean to the right, merely sitting on the Ball will require your body to make adjustments to the left. This automatically strengthens the specific muscles necessary to correct the imbalance.

4. Improves *posture* through strengthening the stabilizing muscles in your torso. As your core muscles become stronger, they will be better able to support your spine in an upright position. This may help to prevent or relieve back pain, because as your spine becomes more elongated, the stress is taken off both your back muscles and the intervertebral discs.

5. Helps develop *body awareness*. As the exercises become more familiar, your focus will shift from an external intellectual process to an internal kinesthetic awareness. Your muscle memory will improve, and you will develop an intuitive

sense of alignment and form. You will feel your body moving as a complete, interconnected mechanism.

6. Evokes *playfulness* and allows you to connect with your inner child. The Ball has the unusual advantage of being fun as well as challenging, which stimulates laughter and creativity and will give you a greater sense of well-being.

7. Provides limited *cardiovascular conditioning.* The Bouncing exercises (see page 68) may provide some degree of aerobic activity, but only if performed for an extended period of time (a minimum of 20 minutes is usually necessary to reach aerobic capacity). Depending on your current level of fitness, your heart rate may not reach your target heart rate zone* during this activity alone. Therefore, in most cases, Bouncing should be used as a warm-up and not as a substitute for cardiovascular activity. **It is recommended that, in addition to the exercises in this book, you do some form of aerobic exercise such as walking, biking or jogging, for 20-60 minutes three times a week.**

* To find your target heart rate zone, subtract your age from the number 220. Then, multiply that number by both 60% and 90% to find the range of beats per minute that you should stay within during any aerobic activity.

The principles developed by Joseph Pilates are integral to your work on the Ball. They impart a sense of mindfulness to every movement, an awareness of being inside your body instead of acting as an observer. There is a strong focus on the quality of each movement, rather than on the number of repetitions or the speed with which they are performed. This keeps your energy in the present and gives you a sense of your body moving as a whole instead of in separate, disconnected parts.

The following six concepts are basic principles in all Pilates®-based training. You will find that, although each one has its own identifiable quality, they are all intrinsically intertwined. Keep these principles in mind as you practice the exercises in this book, but also learn to be aware of them as you move throughout your daily life.

Breathing

Before even beginning a workout, take the time to be still and find your breath. Feel your chest rise and fall, and listen to the sound the air makes as it escapes from your lungs. This will clear your mind and bring your focus into the present moment. You are reminded that your body is alive and your energy level will increase. Be sure to breathe deeply so that your ribcage expands to its fullest as you inhale; then force all the air out as you exhale. As you begin to feel comfortable performing the exercises, allow your breath to coordinate with your movements. Breathing in this manner will provide you with power and momentum, so that your movement can flow more naturally.

Concentration

Stay completely focused on each movement, and try not to let your mind wander. Whenever you notice stray thoughts entering your mind, just let them dissolve, returning your focus to your body and your breathing.

Centering

Once you have found your concentration, center it on a place deep inside the core of your body. This is the place from which all movement grows. Imagine your limbs branching off from your trunk, expanding out into space. Feel a sense of balance in your body between all opposing parts - head and feet, right and left sides, front and back.

Precision

Be precise in the placement of your body, maintaining constant awareness of your alignment and form. There should be no extraneous movements. If you begin to lose this feeling of precision, slow down and bring your focus back to your center.

Control

This is one of the greatest challenges in working on an unstable surface. The Ball sometimes seems to have a mind of its own, but it is inevitable with consistent practice that your movements will become smoother and more controlled. It takes time to build this neuromuscular control, so if you are unable to keep the Ball steady, try an easier variation of the exercise or just continue to practice.

Movement Flow/Rhythm

Every exercise has its own intrinsic rhythm, and this may be different for each individual. Learn to find a comfortable pace that works for your body. You should move carefully so that you can maintain proper form and alignment, but try to give each movement a sense of fluidity and grace.

Many of the exercises in this book have been inspired by specific Mat or Reformer* exercises developed by Joseph Pilates. The Ball exercises, however, are not necessarily *more* effective than traditional Pilates® exercises. Each technique has one basic benefit that the other cannot provide. Much of Joseph Pilates' method uses equipment with springs that provide resistance. Just as with other forms of resistance training - weights, bands and tubing - this will increase your muscle mass faster and to a greater degree than will non-resistive training, especially in the major muscles of your arms and legs. The Ball, on the other hand, provides the element of instability which increases the potential for strengthening the abdominals and other core muscles.

Despite these two significant differences, there are many similar benefits:

O Stretching and strengthening are often combined within the same exercise.

O Stabilization of the spine is important in improving posture and alignment as well as preventing injury.

O The body is strengthened from the inside out, working the muscles closest to the core of the body, then progressing to the larger muscle groups of the extremities.

O Whole body movement is used, often working in more than one range of motion at a time. This is more functional than isolating separate muscle groups.

O Balance is an essential concept. All major muscle groups are strengthened and stretched equally so that there is a sense of symmetry throughout the entire body.

* The Reformer is the most well-known piece of equipment created by Joseph Pilates. It is a wooden frame with a sliding carriage attached to springs which provide resistance.

The Importance of Correct Alignment

The number one reason to strive for correct alignment is injury prevention. When proper alignment is not maintained, there is increased stress on muscles, tendons, ligaments, intervertebral discs, and joint structures. This is the case for all joints in the body, but correct posture of the spine is of special concern. Aside from those injuries caused by traumatic accidents, a large proportion of lower back pain is due to poor posture, which in turn causes repetitive damage or stress. Learning how to find correct posture and strengthening the muscles which support the trunk can help alleviate and prevent lower back soreness or injury by reducing compression on the spinal column and decreasing strain on the back muscles.

There are other benefits to having a stable torso. As your posture improves, you may actually have a feeling of growing taller, and in many cases, there is a measurable increase in height as the spine shifts from a compressed position into an elongated one. Also, strong, stable torso muscles encourage increased mobility in the hip and shoulder joints. For example, if the muscles connecting your pelvis to the rest of your trunk are strong enough to maintain stability while moving your legs, you will then be able to isolate the hip joint and increase its range of motion most effectively.

Having a stable torso does not, however, mean that you must remain in one position all the time. It is essential for a healthy spine to be stretched in a safe range of motion, so moving through a C-curve and an arch are equally important. It is only necessary that neutral spine, a balance between these two extremes, be your natural resting position so as not to put any undue strain on your back.

Spine

To find neutral alignment of the spine, lie on your back with your knees bent and your feet flat on the floor. Try to feel that your spine is as elongated as possible yet very heavy and weighted into the floor. The areas you should feel touching the floor are the back of your pelvis, the back of your ribcage and shoulder blades, and the back of your head. This should create a natural curve in your neck and lower back. Your hip bones should be level with your pubic bone and your head in line with the rest of your body.

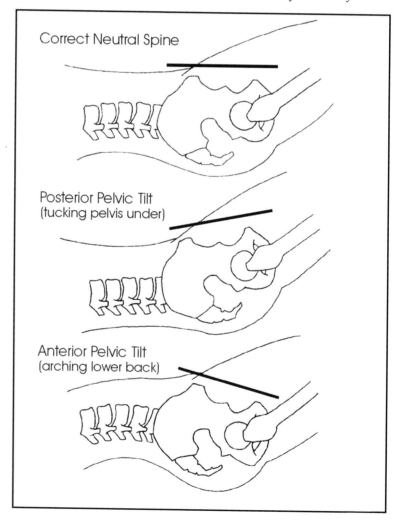

Correct Neutral Spine

Posterior Pelvic Tilt
(tucking pelvis under)

Anterior Pelvic Tilt
(arching lower back)

Shoulder Blades

Engage the shoulder blades by squeezing them together and pulling them downward. This will open out your chest, but be careful not to arch your back at the same time.

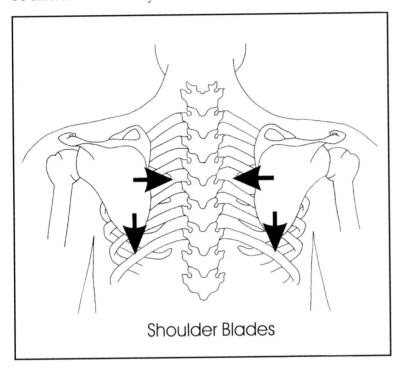

Shoulder Blades

Ribcage and Pelvis

Keep your hips and shoulders square, with the space between your hip bones and ribcage equal on both sides. Unless directed, do not twist or let one side drop lower than the other.

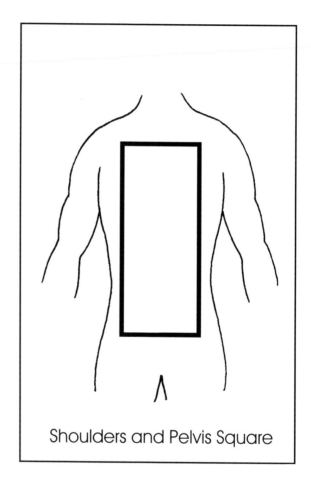

Shoulders and Pelvis Square

Hip and Ankle Joints

Turn out your leg from the hip joint only, not from the knee or ankle. Make sure that your toes always stay in line with your ankle and knee.

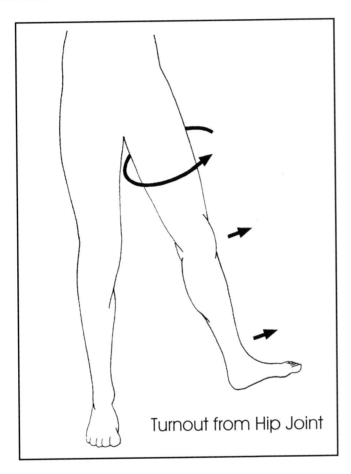

Turnout from Hip Joint

Abdominals and Back

Your abs and back are used in all exercises for stability, so keep your stomach "scooped," or hollowed out and contracted. Imagine that all your abdominal and back muscles are wrapped around your torso like a corset, while pulling your navel in toward your spine.

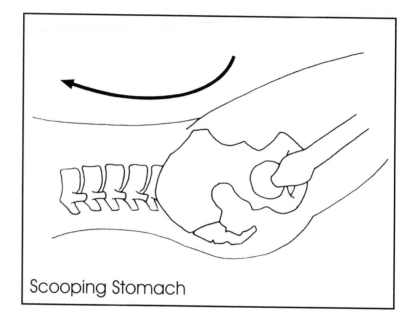

Scooping Stomach

Neutral Spine

Neutral Spine is the natural existing curvature of your spine. This position creates the least stress on the intervertebral discs and the surrounding musculature.

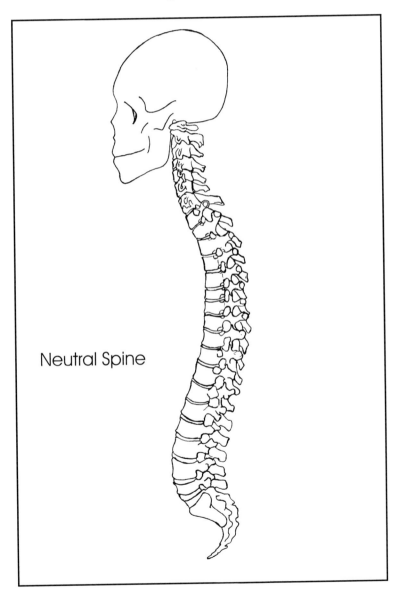

Neutral Spine

C-curve/Arch

A C-curve is a round position of the spine. It involves tucking your pelvis under, bringing your chin to your chest, and hollowing out your stomach. As your spine rounds, your head will come closer to your tailbone. An Arch is a tilting of the pelvis in the opposite direction, as if you are sticking out your tailbone. This creates an increased curve in your lower back, also called hyperextension. An Arch may also involve the upper back and head extending to complete the line of the curve in your lower back. (For example, see Cat Stretch on page 54.)

Prone/Supine

Prone signifies any position lying on your stomach (face down). Supine signifies any position lying on your back (face up).

Turned Out/Turned In/Parallel

To turn out your leg is to rotate your hip joint outward. To turn in your leg is to rotate your hip joint inward. Your leg is in a parallel position when your hip joint is internally rotated just to the point that your knee and foot are aligned with your hip bone. (For examples, see Leg Press on page 90 and Hip Rotation on page 147.)

Flex/Point

To flex your foot is to pull your toes closer to your shin. To point your foot is to stretch your toes away from your shin.

Major Muscle Groups

Because many of these muscle groups work together to perform the same function, this book utilizes three general terms to refer to groups of separate muscles:

1. The rectus abdominis and obliques will be referred to as the *abdominals* when they work collectively to stabilize. The obliques will be mentioned only when they are isolated in twisting or side-bending exercises.

2. The latissimus dorsi, rhomboids, and trapezius will be referred to collectively as the *scapular stabilizers.*

3. The term *hip flexors* will imply use of both the iliopsoas and the quadriceps.

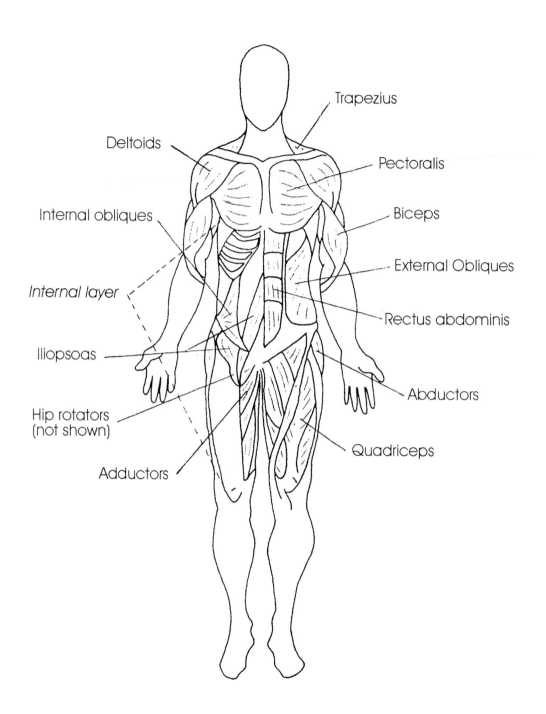

Trapezius

Deltoids

Pectoralis

Internal obliques

Biceps

Internal layer

External Obliques

Iliopsoas

Rectus abdominis

Hip rotators
(not shown)

Abductors

Adductors

Quadriceps

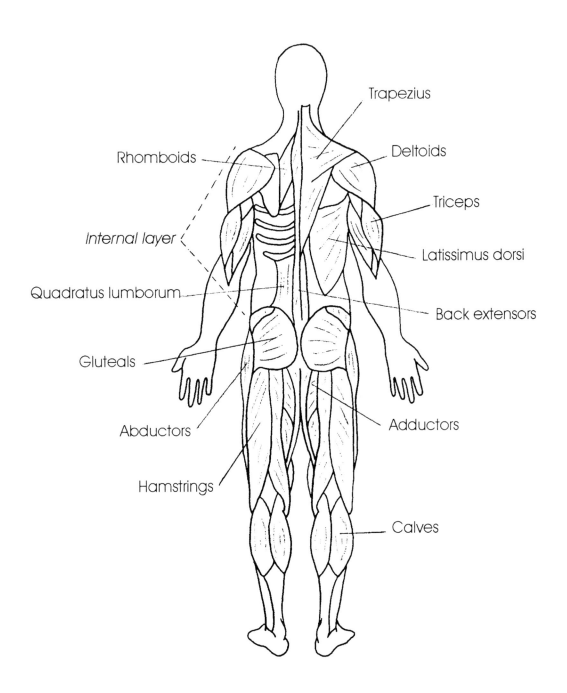

Trapezius

Rhomboids

Deltoids

Triceps

Internal layer

Latissimus dorsi

Quadratus lumborum

Back extensors

Gluteals

Abductors

Adductors

Hamstrings

Calves

Choosing the Right Size Ball

When sitting on the Ball, your knees should be at a 90° angle or just slightly lower than the level of your hips. Following are some general guidelines based on your height; however, you may wish to choose a different size Ball depending on the proportion of your legs to your torso (i.e. longer legs may necessitate a larger Ball). If in doubt, choose a larger size Ball so that you may under-inflate it.

5' to 5'6"	55 cm
5'7" to 6'2"	65 cm
over 6'2"	75 cm

Note: You may find it desirable to under-inflate your Ball in the beginning when it is the most firm. Over time your Ball will likely gain elasticity and become softer. When this happens, you may need to add more air to reach the preferred height while seated.

Getting Started

The exercises in this book are divided into three levels that are indicated with the following symbols:

Beginner   O

Intermediate   OO

Advanced   OOO

It is recommended that you start with the Beginner exercises and progress to more difficult ones only when you feel completely ready. Before attempting an exercise, please read the whole movement description thoroughly. Included with each strengthening exercise is a suggested number of repetitions. Because the stretches should be held as long as they are comfortable, many only need to be performed once. Variations are given when an exercise can be done in different positions to increase the level of difficulty or to work different muscle groups. Also provided are a list of the major muscle groups being strengthened and some helpful tips to maintain correct alignment and form.

To help you get started, three sample workouts are included in the back of the book, but they are by no means all-inclusive. They are merely guidelines, so feel free to adapt them to the needs of your body. You may replace certain exercises with others that work similar muscle groups or add any that are particularly fun or challenging, as long as you strive to design a thorough, balanced workout that stretches and strengthens every major muscle group in the body.

Chapter One: Lying/Sitting on the Floor

Footwork on the Wall

Roll Up

Lie on your back with your knees bent and your feet flat on the floor, hip-width apart. Place the Ball on your thighs, gently resting your hands on the Ball. Keeping your arms straight, raise your head and upper back off the floor into a stomach crunch. Hold this position for a few seconds, then lower your head back down to the floor. ○

Suggested Repetitions: 10

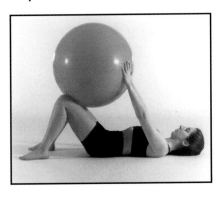 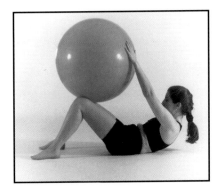

Variation #1: Place one hand behind your head and raise your head and chest up toward that side, keeping your elbow on the floor. ○

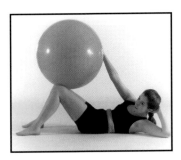

TIPS

✓ The Ball will roll up toward your knees as you lift your upper body off the floor. This movement should be a result only of the abdominals working to raise your torso, not of your shoulders hunching forward or your elbows bending and straightening.

MAJOR MUSCLE GROUPS

♦ abdominals
♦ obliques (Variation #1)

Basic: Lie on your back with your feet resting on top of the Ball. Your legs should be straight and in a parallel position. Bend and straighten your legs, rolling the Ball back and forth in a straight line. ○
Suggested Repetitions: 10

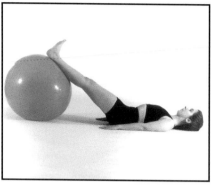
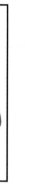
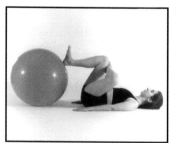

Variation #1: Keep your legs turned out and your heels together. ○

Variation #2: Cross one foot over the opposite knee. ○

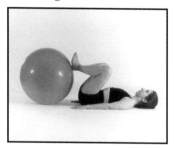

Stomach Crunch: Place your hands behind your head and raise your head and upper back off the floor into a stomach crunch. Hold this position and repeat the Basic Footwork. Keep your elbows wide. ○
Suggested Repetitions: 10

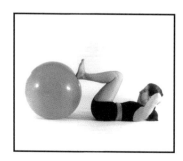

Variation #1: Keep your legs turned out and your heels together. ○

Variation #2: Cross one foot over the opposite knee. ○

Twist: Place your hands behind your head and raise your torso up toward one side. Hold this position and repeat the Basic Footwork. Keep your elbows wide with one elbow remaining on the floor as the other lifts up. Repeat on the other side. ○
Suggested Repetitions: 10 each side

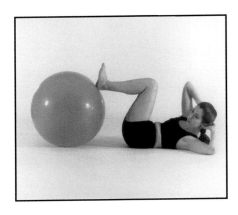

Variation #1: Keep your legs turned out and your heels together. ○

Double Leg Stretch: Repeat the Stomach Crunch Footwork, beginning with your knees bent and your hands on your shins. As you straighten your legs, raise your arms overhead to the level of your face. As you bend your knees, circle your arms around to the side and back to your shins. Keep your head and upper back lifted off the floor the entire time. ○
Suggested Repetitions: 10

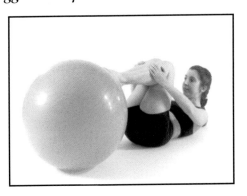 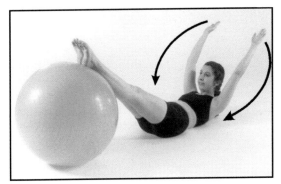

Single Leg Stretch: Begin in the Stomach Crunch position, with your right foot on the Ball, leg straight, and your left knee bent in toward your chest. From there, bend your right leg and straighten your left leg just above the Ball. Then, as you straighten your right leg, bend your left knee in toward your chest. The Ball rolls back and forth under your right foot. Repeat on the other side. ○

Suggested Repetitions: 10 sets each side

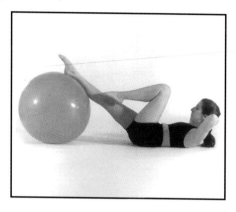 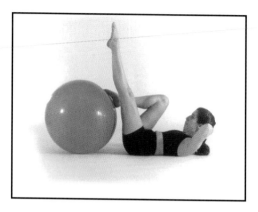

Criss-Cross: Repeat the Single Leg Stretch, reaching your elbow toward the opposite knee to work the obliques. Keep your elbows wide with one elbow remaining on the floor as the other lifts up. Repeat on the other side. ○

Suggested Repetitions: 10 sets each side

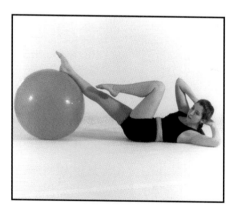 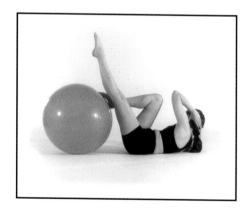

TIPS

✓ Always try to roll the Ball back and forth in a completely straight line.

✓ When you are holding a stomach crunch position, make sure that your whole upper back is raised off the floor, except for the very tip of each shoulder blade which should still be down.

✓ Keep your tailbone on the floor.

✓ When both feet are on the Ball, focus on squeezing your inner thighs together.

MAJOR MUSCLE GROUPS

♦ abdominals

♦ hamstrings

♦ quadriceps

♦ adductors

♦ obliques (Twist and Criss-Cross)

♦ hip rotators (Variation #1)

Stretch for: gluteals (Variation #2)

Shoulder Bridge

Basic: Lie on your back and rest your legs on top of the Ball, knees bent. Tuck your pelvis under and press your hips up toward the ceiling, rolling one vertebra at a time. Then roll your hips back down to the floor, one vertebra at a time. Try to keep the Ball steady. ○
Suggested Repetitions: 8

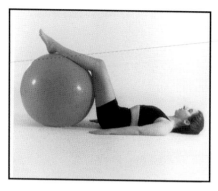 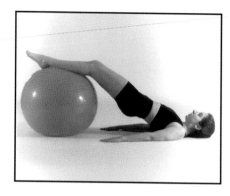

Straight Leg Bridge: Place your feet on top of the Ball and repeat the Basic Shoulder Bridge. Keep your legs straight and in a parallel position. ○
Suggested Repetitions: 8

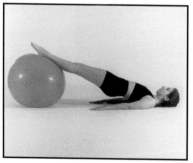

Variation #1: Keep your legs turned out and your heels together. ○

Variation #2: Cross one leg over the other. ○

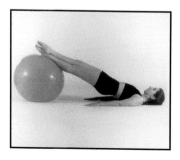

Leg Lifts: Begin in the Basic Shoulder Bridge position. Lift one leg off the Ball and try to hold your balance for at least 5 seconds. Repeat on the other side. ○
Suggested Repetitions: 4 sets

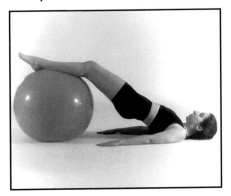 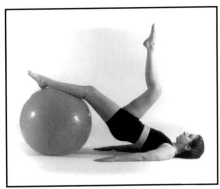

Variation #1: Begin in the Straight Leg Bridge position. ○

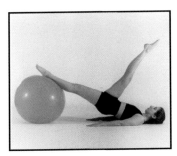

Variation #2: Begin in the Straight Leg Bridge position. Lift one leg off the Ball, touch your toes to the opposite knee, straighten your leg back up to the ceiling, and lower down to the Ball. ○○

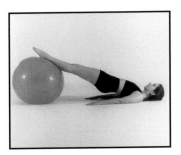 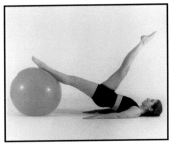 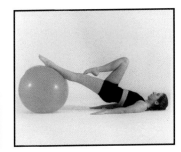

Variation #3: Begin in the Straight Leg Bridge position. Lift one leg off the Ball and carry it sideways across your body. The Ball will roll slightly in the opposite direction. Bring your leg back to vertical and lower down to the Ball. ○○

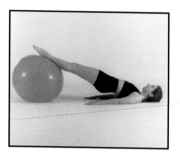 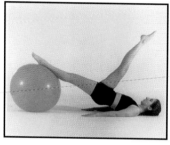 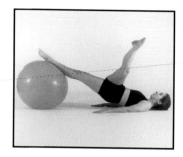

Leg Curl: Begin in the Straight Leg Bridge position. Keep your hips pressed high while bending and straightening your legs. The Ball will roll in toward your hips as you bend your knees. ○○
Suggested Repetitions: 8

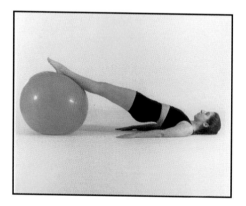 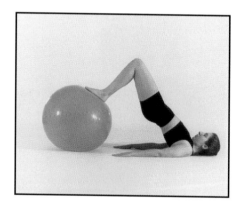

Variation #1: Keep your legs turned out and your heels together. ○○

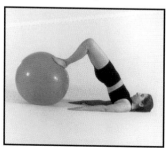

Single Leg Curl: Begin in the Straight Leg Bridge position. Keeping your right leg straight, bend your left knee in toward your chest. From there, bend and straighten your legs in opposition. The Ball rolls back and forth under your right foot (see Single Leg Stretch on page 34). Repeat on the other side. ○○○
Suggested Repetitions: 4 sets each side

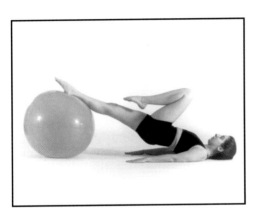 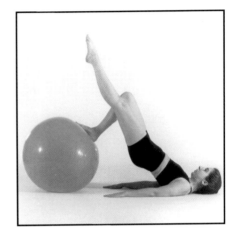

TIPS
✓ When rolling through your back, articulate each vertebra in the spinal column.

✓ Keep your buttocks and abdominals tight.

✓ When one leg is lifted up, try to keep your hips square.

✓ Raise one or both of your arms up toward the ceiling to make it more difficult to balance.

MAJOR MUSCLE GROUPS
♦ abdominals

♦ back extensors

♦ hamstrings

♦ gluteals

♦ hip rotators (Straight Leg Bridge Variation #1 and Leg Curl Variation #1)

Stretch for: hip flexors (Leg Curl)

Roll Over

Knee Extension (Preparation): Lie on your back with the Ball between your ankles and your knees bent. Straighten your legs up toward the ceiling, then bend your knees until the Ball touches the floor. Keep your tailbone on the floor the entire time. ◯
Suggested Repetitions: 10

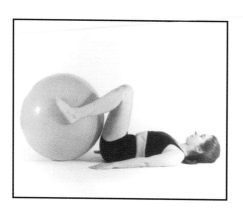
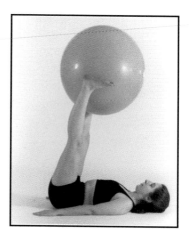

Hip Lift (Preparation): Lie on your back with the Ball between your ankles and your legs straight up toward the ceiling. From there, lift your hips off the floor just a few inches. Try to keep your legs vertical instead of rocking them overhead. ◯
Suggested Repetitions: 10

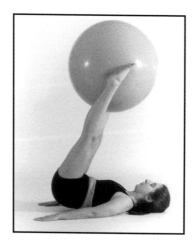

Roll Over: Lie on your back with the Ball between your ankles and your knees bent. Straighten your legs up toward the ceiling, then lift your hips off the floor to roll over, bringing your legs overhead. Try to touch the Ball to the floor behind you. From there, roll your back down one vertebra at a time until your legs are vertical, then bend your knees until the Ball touches the floor. ○○
Suggested Repetitions: 5-8

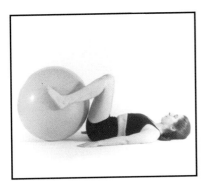
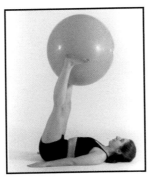
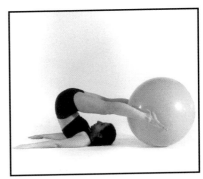

Variation #1: Repeat the Roll Over, but when your legs are overhead, take the Ball in your hands and roll down. The second time, when your legs are overhead, place the Ball between your ankles and roll down again. ○○

Jack-knife: Repeat the Roll Over, but once the Ball is overhead, lift your legs up even higher into a shoulder stand. From there, lower your legs overhead to touch the Ball to the floor and roll down. ○○○
Suggested Repetitions: 4-5

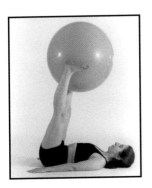
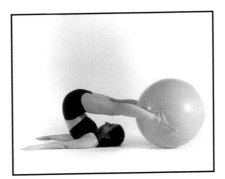
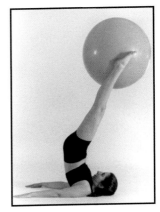

Variation #1: Bypass the Roll Over position and lift your legs straight up to the shoulder stand. ○○○

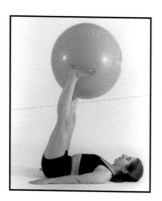 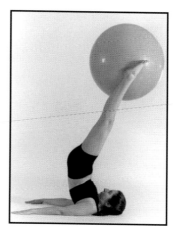

TIPS

✓ Do not arch your back as you bend and straighten your legs.

✓ Roll through your back sequentially and make sure that your tailbone touches the floor before you bend your knees.

MAJOR MUSCLE GROUPS

- ◆ abdominals
- ◆ hip flexors
- ◆ adductors
- ◆ quadriceps (Knee Extension)
- ◆ gluteals (Jack-knife)
- ◆ back extensors (Jack-knife)

Stretch for: hamstrings, back extensors (Roll Over)

Corkscrew

Lie on your back with the Ball between your ankles and your legs straight up toward the ceiling. Circle both legs in a clockwise direction, all the way around and back to vertical. Repeat alternating directions. ○

Suggested Repetitions: 4 sets

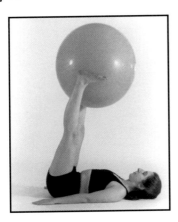 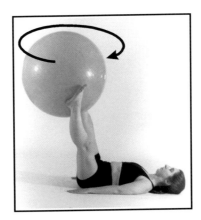

TIPS

✓ Keep the circles small so that your tailbone stays on the floor and your hips remain stable.

✓ Make the circles smooth, as if you are passing through every point around the face of a clock.

✓ Keep your lower back pressed into the floor the entire time.

✓ You may bend your legs slightly to prevent any tension in the quadriceps.

MAJOR MUSCLE GROUPS

♦ abdominals
♦ hip flexors
♦ adductors

Stretch for: hamstrings

Leg Twist

Lie on your back with the Ball between your ankles and your legs straight up toward the ceiling. Twist the Ball so that your right leg crosses over the left. Bring the Ball back to the center, then twist the other direction. ○

Suggested Repetitions: 4 sets

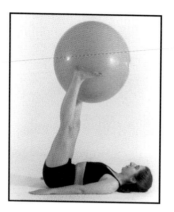 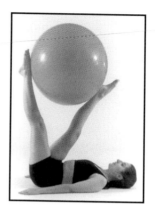

TIPS
   ✓ Keep your lower back pressed into the floor the entire time.
   ✓ Your pelvis should remain stable.

MAJOR MUSCLE GROUPS
   ◆ abdominals
   ◆ adductors
   ◆ hip flexors
   Stretch for: hamstrings

Toss and Catch

Lie on your back with your legs in the air, holding the Ball in your hands. Throw the Ball up into the air and try to catch it between your ankles. From there, let the Ball fall back into your hands as your legs open gently to the side. ○

Suggested Repetitions: 10

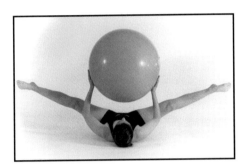 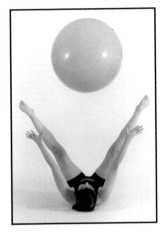 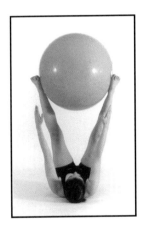

TIPS

✓ Keep your lower back pressed into the floor the entire time.

✓ Your pelvis should remain stable.

✓ If possible, keep your legs straight.

✓ Your legs should open and close in a flat, vertical plane. Try not to let them move too far away from you.

MAJOR MUSCLE GROUPS

♦ abdominals

♦ adductors

♦ hip flexors

♦ biceps

♦ triceps

♦ pectoralis

Stretch for: hamstrings, adductors

Torso Twist

Basic: Lie on your back with your knees bent in toward your chest. Hold the Ball in your hands, arms straight up toward the ceiling. From there, simultaneously lower the Ball to your right and your knees to your left. Do not let your knees touch the floor. Then, using your abdominals, bring your knees and the Ball back to the center. Repeat on the other side. ○
Suggested Repetitions: 4 sets

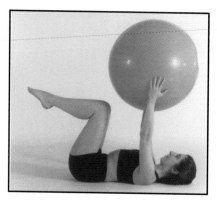 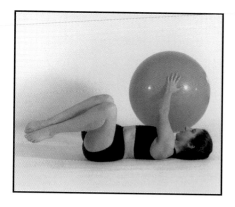

Torso Stretch: Lie on your back with your knees bent and your feet flat on the floor. Hold the Ball in your hands, arms straight up toward the ceiling. From there, simultaneously lower the Ball to your right and your knees to your left, letting your legs relax completely. Then, using your abdominals, bring your knees and the Ball back to the center. Repeat on the other side. ○

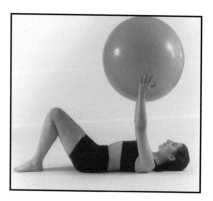 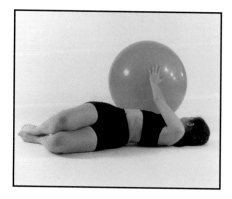

TIPS

✓ By keeping your legs off the floor in the Basic Torso Twist, you are ensuring that the correct muscles are working.

✓ Use the Ball for resistance and balance.

MAJOR MUSCLE GROUPS

♦ obliques

Stretch for: abductors, back extensors, obliques

Hamstring Stretch

Lie on your back and rest your legs on the Ball, knees bent. Straighten one leg up toward the ceiling, holding either your thigh or ankle, and pull your leg in toward your chest to stretch the hamstrings. Repeat on the other side. ○

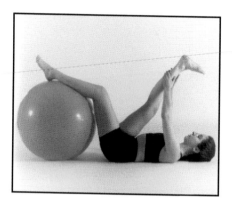

Variation #1: While you are stretching, gently circle your ankle in both directions. ○

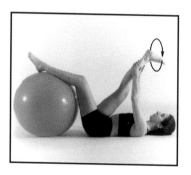

Variation #2: Bend and straighten your leg with your foot flexed, pulling your leg in a little closer each time you straighten. ○

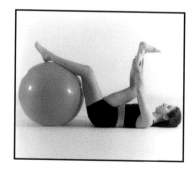

Variation #3: Hold your leg with the opposite hand and pull across your body to stretch the outer thigh. Let the Ball roll slightly to counterbalance. ○

Variation #4: Hold your leg with the same hand and let your leg open out to the side to stretch the inner thigh. You may rest your leg on the floor, letting the opposite hip lift up as needed. ○

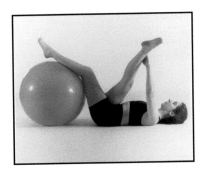
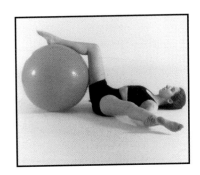

TIPS
✓ Make sure your tailbone stays on the floor (except for Variation #4).

MAJOR MUSCLE GROUPS
Stretch for: hamstrings, calves (Variations #1 & #2), abductors (Variation #3), adductors (Variation #4)

Teaser

Lie on your back with your feet on top of the Ball, your legs straight, and your arms resting on the floor above your head. In one smooth motion, sit up and reach your arms forward on a high diagonal. From there, raise your arms up to the level of your face and roll back down to the floor, one vertebra at a time. ◯◯

Suggested Repetitions: 4-5

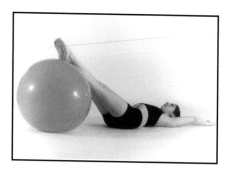
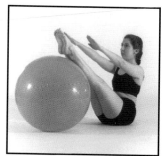
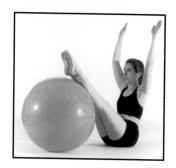

TIPS

✓ As you roll down, try to keep your arms in place above your head. If you have difficulty rolling down with control, you may reach them forward to help counterbalance.

MAJOR MUSCLE GROUPS

♦ abdominals

♦ hip flexors

Stretch for: hamstrings

Reverse Flat Back

Begin sitting on the floor with your feet resting on top of the Ball and your legs straight. Place your hands behind you with your fingers pointing away from the Ball. From there, press your hips up toward the ceiling until your body is in a straight line. Hold this position for a few seconds, then lower your hips back down to the floor. ○○○

Suggested Repetitions: 4-5

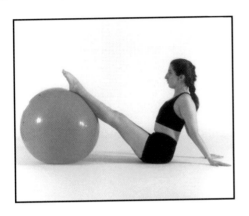
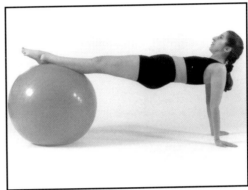

TIPS
✓ Keep your buttocks and abdominals tight.
✓ Your focus should remain forward.
✓ Do not lock your elbows.

MAJOR MUSCLE GROUPS
♦ abdominals
♦ back extensors
♦ hamstrings
♦ gluteals
♦ scapular stabilizers
Stretch for: deltoids

Side Kicks

Knee Extension: Lie on the floor on your left side with your left leg slightly in front of you at an angle. Place your right foot on top of the Ball with your leg straight out to the side, turned out. Prop your head up in your left hand. From there, bend and straighten your right leg, rolling the Ball back and forth in a straight line. Repeat on the other side. ○
Suggested Repetitions: 8 each side

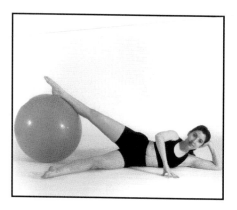 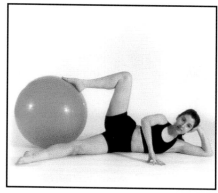

Hip Rotation: Lie on the floor on your left side with your left leg slightly in front of you at an angle. Place your right foot on top of the Ball with your leg turned out, knee bent. Prop your head up in your left hand. From there, rotate your right leg in and out, rolling the Ball back and forth just slightly. Repeat on the other side. ○
Suggested Repetitions: 8 each side

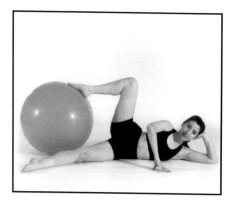 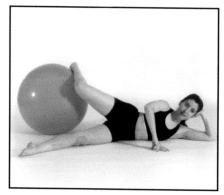

TIPS

✓ Keep your hips square to the front.

✓ Keep your working leg turned out the entire time in the Knee Extension.

MAJOR MUSCLE GROUPS

- ♦ abdominals
- ♦ back extensors
- ♦ quadriceps
- ♦ hamstrings
- ♦ hip rotators

Stretch for: adductors

Cat Stretch

Kneel with your hands on the Ball and your spine in a C-curve. Do not sit back all the way onto your heels. From there, arch your back and look up toward the ceiling. The Ball may roll forward just slightly. ○
Suggested Repetitions: 8

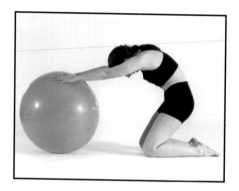 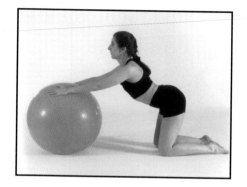

TIPS

✓ In the C-curve, you should have very little weight on your hands. When you arch, press your hands onto the Ball to engage the triceps. Keep your arms straight the entire time.

✓ When you arch your back, keep your spine in a long, curved line from your head to your tailbone, being careful not to compress the vertebrae in either your lower back or neck.

MAJOR MUSCLE GROUPS

♦ abdominals
♦ back extensors
♦ triceps
♦ scapular stabilizers

Stretch for: abdominals, back extensors

Footwork on the Wall

Basic: Lie on your back with your knees bent in toward your chest. Place the Ball against the wall supported by both of your feet. Keeping your legs together, bend and straighten your legs, rolling the Ball up and down on the wall. ❍

Suggested Repetitions: 8

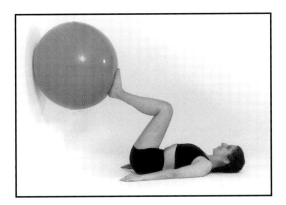
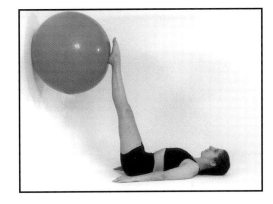

Variation #1:
Keep your legs turned out and your heels together. ❍

Variation #2:
Cross one foot over the opposite knee. ❍

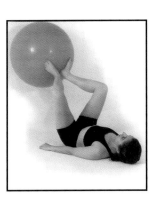
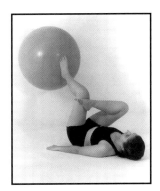

Variation #3: Straighten your free leg up toward the ceiling. ○

Variation #4: Straighten your free leg out to your side, keeping both hips on the floor and your working leg in a parallel position. ○

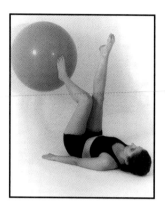
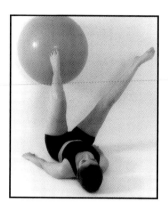

Stomach Crunch: Place your hands behind your head and raise your head and upper back off the floor into a stomach crunch. Hold this position and repeat the Basic Footwork on the Wall. Keep your elbows wide. ○
Suggested Repetitions: 8

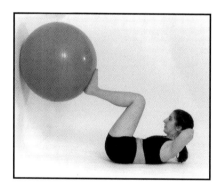

Variation #1: Keep your legs turned out and your heels together. ○

Variation #2: Cross one foot over the opposite knee. ○

Variation #3: Straighten your free leg up toward the ceiling. ○

Variation #4: Straighten your free leg out to your side, keeping both hips on the floor and your working leg in a parallel position. ○

Side Kicks: Lie on the floor on your left side with your left leg straight, your foot touching the wall. Place the Ball against the wall supported by your right foot, keeping your leg turned out, knee bent. Prop your head up in your left hand. From there, bend and straighten your right leg, rolling the Ball up and down on the wall. Repeat on the other side. ◯

Suggested Repetitions: 8 each side

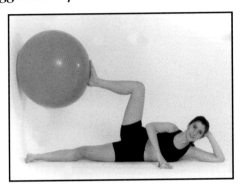 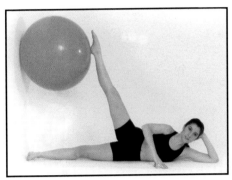

Variation #1: Keep your bottom leg lifted off the floor a few inches. ◯

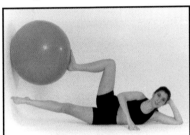

TIPS

✓ You will need to adjust your starting position for the Basic Footwork on the Wall so that your tailbone stays on the floor the entire time.

✓ Try to roll the Ball in a straight line.

MAJOR MUSCLE GROUPS

♦ abdominals
♦ quadriceps
♦ hamstrings
♦ hip rotators (Basic/Stomach Crunch Variation #1 and Side Kicks)
♦ adductors (Basic/Stomach Crunch Variation #4 and Side Kicks Variation #1)

Stretch for: hamstrings, gluteals (Variation #2), adductors (Side Kicks)

Chapter Two: Sitting on the Ball

Pelvic Tilts

Front to Back: Sit on the Ball with your feet flat on the floor, hip-width apart. Isolating the hips, tuck the pelvis under, then return to neutral. Next, tilt the pelvis to arch the lower back, then return to neutral. ○

Suggested Repetitions: 8 sets

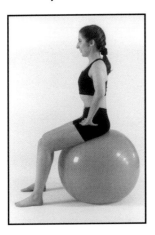 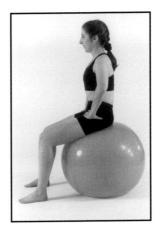 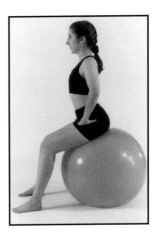

Variation #1: Tilt the pelvis front to back without pausing in neutral. ○

Variation #2: Place your feet as wide as possible with your legs turned out. ○

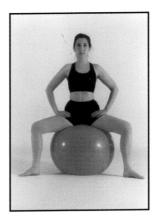

Side to Side: Sit on the Ball with your feet flat on the floor, hip-width apart. Isolating the hips, tilt the pelvis to one side, then return to neutral. Repeat alternating sides. ○
Suggested Repetitions: 8 sets

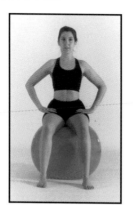 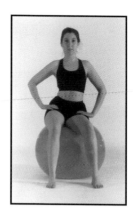

Variation #1: Tilt the pelvis side to side without pausing in neutral. ○

Variation #2: Place your feet as wide as possible with your legs turned out. ○

Circles: Sit on the Ball with your feet flat on the floor, hip-width apart. Isolating the hips, move the pelvis in a circle, tilting to the front, to the right, to the back, and to the left. Repeat reversing the direction. ○
Suggested Repetitions: 8 each direction

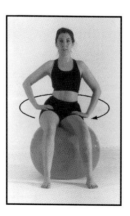

Variation #1: Smooth out the circle so that you do not pause in each position. ○

Variation #2: Place your feet as wide as possible with your legs turned out. ○

TIPS

✓ Sit up tall, keeping your shoulders level and your spine in a neutral position from the waist up.

✓ Your torso should remain still to isolate the pelvis.

✓ Placing your feet closer together will make it more difficult to keep your balance.

MAJOR MUSCLE GROUPS

♦ abdominals
♦ back extensors (Front to Back and Circles)
♦ obliques (Side to Side and Circles)
♦ quadratus lumborum (Side to Side and Circles)
♦ abductors (Variation #2)

Stretch for: adductors (Variation #2)

Leg Lifts

Basic: Begin sitting on the Ball with your feet together. Lift one foot off the floor, keeping your knee bent. Try to hold your balance for at least 5 seconds. Repeat on the other side. ◯

Suggested Repetitions: 4 sets

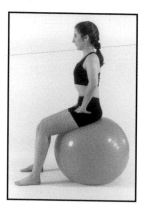

Variation #1: Straighten your leg as you lift it up. ◯

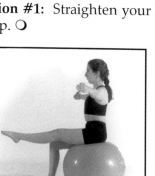

Variation #2: Circle the ankle as you hold your balance. ◯

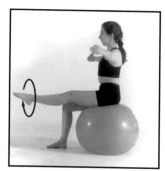

Twist: Begin sitting on the Ball with your feet together and your arms out to the side. Lift your left leg, twist your torso to your left, return back to the center and lower your leg. Repeat on the other side. ○

Suggested Repetitions: 4 sets

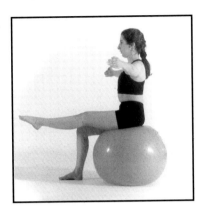
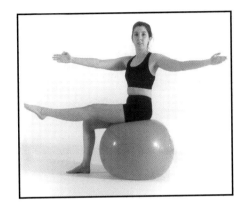

TIPS

✓ Do not sink into your hips or let your pelvis tuck under. Instead, sit up as tall as possible and keep your spine in a neutral position.

✓ Extend your arms out to the side to help balance.

✓ Place your feet hip-width apart to make it more challenging.

MAJOR MUSCLE GROUPS

♦ abdominals

♦ back extensors

♦ hip flexors

♦ obliques (Twist)

Forward Roll

Sit on the Ball with your feet flat on the floor, hip-width apart. Keep your spine in a neutral position as you roll the Ball forward and back, as if you are sitting in a chair on wheels. ❍
Suggested Repetitions: 10

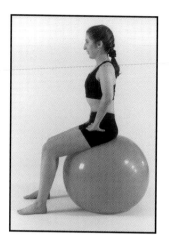 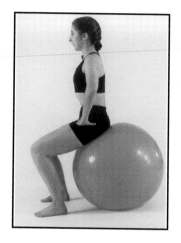

Variation #1: Place your feet close together. ❍

Variation #2: Raise your heels off the floor, keeping your legs together. ❍

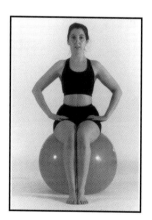 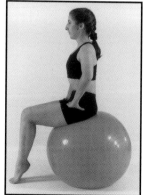

Variation #3: Cross your ankles so that only your toes are on the floor. ○

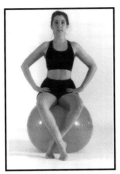

Variation #4: Lift one foot off the floor, extending the leg forward. ○

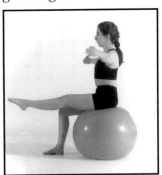

Variation #5: Cross one foot over the opposite knee. ○○

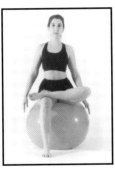

TIPS

✓ You may need to begin with your feet a little farther away from the Ball to provide more room to roll.

✓ Keep your torso completely still. You should be moving only at the knee joint.

✓ Extend your arms out to the side to help balance.

MAJOR MUSCLE GROUPS

♦ abdominals
♦ back extensors
♦ quadriceps
♦ hamstrings
♦ calves (Variation #2)
♦ hip rotators (Variation #3)
♦ hip flexors (Variation #4)
Stretch for: gluteals (Variation #5)

Basic: Sit on the Ball with your feet flat on the floor, hip-width apart. Bounce up and down, keeping your spine in a neutral position and your feet on the floor the entire time. ○
Suggested Repetitions: 20-40

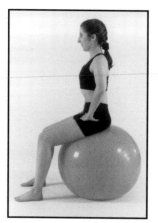 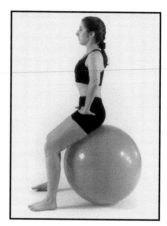

Variation #1: Bounce using your feet to push off the floor. Be sure to roll through your feet toe-ball-heel. ○

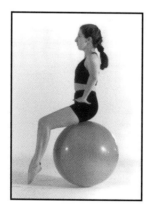

Variation #2: Bounce with one leg lifted off the floor. ○

Variation #3: Place your feet as wide as possible with your legs turned out. ○

Pelvic Tilts: Sit on the Ball with your feet flat on the floor, hip-width apart. Bounce up and down, tilting your pelvis front and back, side to side, or in a circle (see Pelvic Tilts on page 61). Make sure that your pelvis tilts only as your hips lift up off the Ball. Your spine should return to neutral as you bounce down on the Ball to prevent compression of the discs. Keep your feet on the floor the entire time. ❍❍

Suggested Repetitions: 8 sets of each

Jumping Jacks: Sit on the Ball with your feet flat on the floor, hip-width apart. Bounce up and down with your feet moving together and apart, raising your arms up and down to the side. ❍❍

Suggested Repetitions: 10

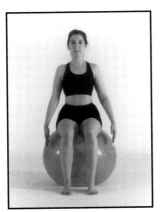 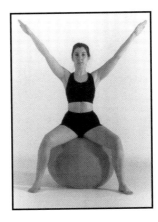

Russian Kicks: Sit on the Ball with your feet flat on the floor, hip-width apart. Bounce up and down from one leg to the other, kicking your free leg forward. Keep your arms crossed in front of your chest. ❍❍

Suggested Repetitions: 10 sets

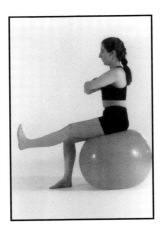

TIPS

✓ Practice bouncing at various speeds, so that you are using the muscles in your legs to control the movement. The slower the tempo, the more the legs have to work.

✓ Keep your spine vertical, especially as you bounce more slowly.

✓ Press your heels into the floor as you bounce to help keep your center of gravity over the Ball.

MAJOR MUSCLE GROUPS

♦ quadriceps
♦ gluteals
♦ abdominals
♦ calves (Variation #1)
♦ abductors (Variation #3)
♦ deltoids (Jumping Jacks)

Hinge

Basic: Sit on the Ball with your feet flat on the floor, hip-width apart, and your hands behind your head. From there, hinge backward from the hip joint to a slight diagonal, and then return to vertical. Try to keep your back completely flat like a board. ○
Suggested Repetitions: 5-8

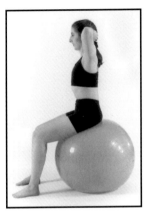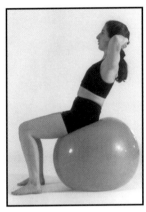

Twist: Sit on the Ball with your feet flat on the floor, hip-width apart, and your hands behind your head. From there, twist to your left, hinge backward from the hip joint to a slight diagonal, return to vertical, and twist back to the center. Repeat on the other side. ○
Suggested Repetitions: 3-4 sets

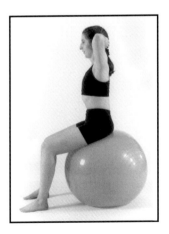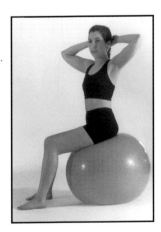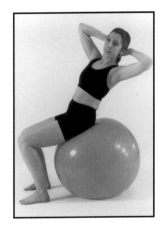

TIPS

✓ Be especially careful not to arch your back as you hinge.

✓ When you lean back in a twist, keep the space between your ribcage and hip bones equidistant on both sides.

✓ Keep your elbows wide.

✓ The Ball may roll forward slightly as you hinge.

MAJOR MUSCLE GROUPS

♦ abdominals
♦ back extensors
♦ hip flexors
♦ obliques (Twist)

Straddle

Basic: Sit straddling the Ball with your knees on the sides and your toes on the floor behind you. From there, squeeze your inner thighs against the Ball and release. ⭕
Suggested Repetitions: 10

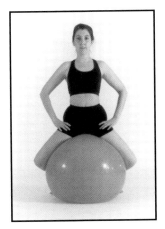

Side Stretch: Sit straddling the Ball with your knees on the sides and your toes on the floor behind you. With both arms raised overhead, tilt your torso to the right so that you feel a stretch along the left side of your body. The Ball will shift slightly to the left. Repeat on the other side. ⭕⭕
Suggested Repetitions: 2 sets

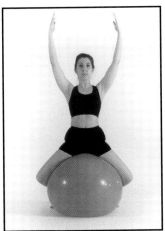 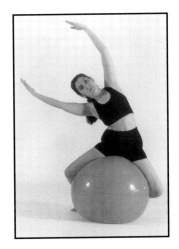

Arch: Sit straddling the Ball with your knees on the sides and your toes on the floor behind you. With both arms raised overhead, arch your back slightly, taking your focus up toward the ceiling. Then bring your spine back to neutral. ○○○
Suggested Repetitions: 4

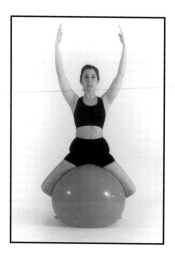 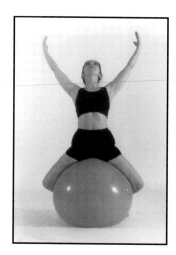

TIPS

✓ When you arch, lift up out of your hips and keep your pelvis tucked under to protect your lower back. Focus on arching your upper back rather than your lower back.

✓ The farther apart you place your feet, the easier it will be to balance.

MAJOR MUSCLE GROUPS

♦ abdominals
♦ adductors
♦ obliques (Side Stretch)
♦ back extensors (Arch)

Stretch for: adductors, hip flexors, obliques (Side Stretch), abdominals and pectoralis (Arch)

Hamstring/Back Stretch

Sit on the Ball with your feet flat on the floor, hip-width apart (or wider if it is more comfortable). Round your back forward to hang all the way over, rolling the Ball backward slightly to straighten your legs. As your legs straighten, flex your feet to get an additional stretch in your calves. ○

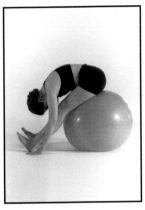

Variation #1: Rock back and forth, gently bending and straightening your knees. ○

Variation #2: Clasp your hands behind your back and stretch your arms up toward the ceiling. ○

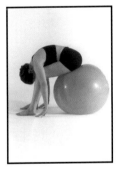 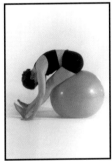 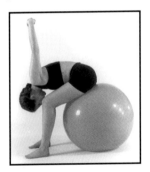

TIPS
✓ Let your head and neck relax completely.

MAJOR MUSCLE GROUPS
♦ abdominals

Stretch for: hamstrings, back extensors, calves, pectoralis and deltoids (Variation #2)

Gluteal Stretch

Sit on the Ball with one foot crossed over the opposite knee. Then round your back forward to hang over your leg. Let your arms hang freely, reaching toward the floor. You may keep the supporting leg bent or roll back slightly to straighten. Repeat on the other side. ◐○

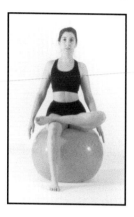 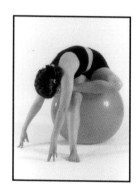

Variation #1: Rock back and forth, gently bending and straightening your knee. ◐○

Variation #2: Reach your hands toward the floor on the side of the supporting leg. ◐○

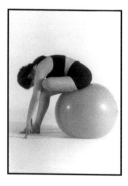 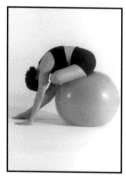 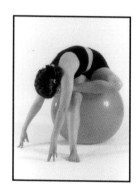

TIPS

✓ It may be easier to touch the floor, and thereby keep your balance, with the supporting leg straight.

MAJOR MUSCLE GROUPS

♦ abdominals

Stretch for: gluteals, back extensors, hamstrings, quadratus lumborum (Variation #2)

Seated Side Stretch

Sit on the Ball and place your feet as wide as possible with your legs turned out. Keeping your left leg bent and your right leg straight, stretch over to the right while reaching your left arm overhead. Repeat on the other side. ❍

Suggested Repetitions: 2 sets

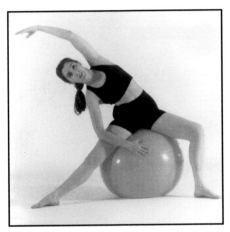

TIPS

✓ Keep your shoulders and hips square to the front so that your torso does not twist.

MAJOR MUSCLE GROUPS

♦ abdominals
♦ obliques

Stretch for: obliques, adductors, hamstrings

Chapter Three: Lying on the Ball (Supine)

Stomach Crunch

Basic: Begin sitting on the Ball with your feet flat on the floor, hip-width apart. With your hands behind your head, walk your feet forward until your lower back is resting on the Ball. Contracting the abdominals, raise and lower the upper half of your torso. The range of motion is short, keeping your spine in a C-curve. ○

Suggested Repetitions: 10

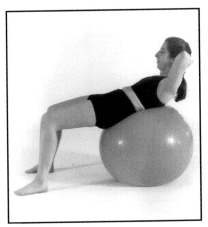 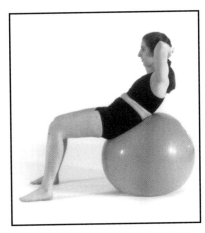

Variation #1: To work the obliques, curl up on a diagonal toward one knee. Repeat alternating sides. ○

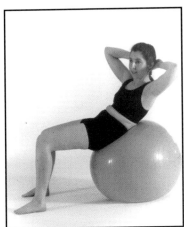

Pulses: Begin sitting on the Ball with your feet flat on the floor, hip-width apart. Walk your feet forward until your lower back is resting on the Ball. Reach your arms forward and pulse your torso up in very small movements. ○
Suggested Repetitions: 10

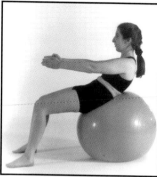

Variation #1: Reach your arms toward one knee and pulse your torso up, contracting the obliques on the side you are twisting toward. ○

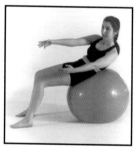

TIPS

✓ Keep your elbows wide.

✓ Your pelvis stays tucked under, and the upper half of your torso (from the ribcage to the head) moves in one piece, as if in a body cast.

✓ Do not let your upper back collapse onto the Ball or allow your lower back to arch.

✓ For the Basic Variation #1, reach your shoulder, rather than your elbow, up toward your knee. Imagine that you are folding your whole torso in half diagonally.

✓ The Pulses are smaller and slightly quicker than the Basic Stomach Crunch.

MAJOR MUSCLE GROUPS

♦ abdominals

♦ obliques (Variation #1)

Flat Back

Basic: Begin sitting on the Ball with your feet flat on the floor, hip-width apart and your arms reaching forward. Walk your feet forward until only your shoulders and head are resting on the Ball, raising your arms overhead simultaneously. Keep your hips pressed up toward the ceiling, so they are in line with your knees and shoulders. From there, walk your feet in, bringing your torso back to vertical and your arms forward. ○
Suggested Repetitions: 5-8

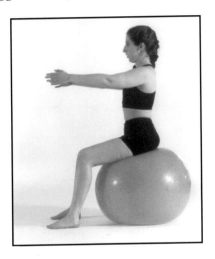 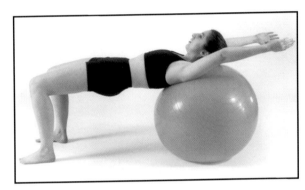

Pulses: Begin in the Basic Flat Back position. Slowly pulse your hips up toward the ceiling. This movement is very small, just a repeated contraction of the gluteals. ○
Suggested Repetitions: 10

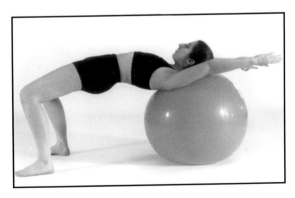

Heel Raises: Begin in the Basic Flat Back position. Lift your heels off the floor so that you are balancing on the balls of your feet, then place them back down on the floor. ○
Suggested Repetitions: 10

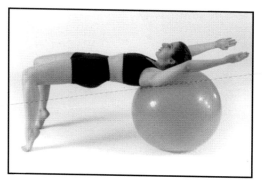

Quad Stretch: Begin in the Basic Flat Back position. Bring one foot in closer to the Ball so that you feel a stretch in the front of your thigh. Your heel may lift off the floor slightly. Keep your hips lifted and your pelvis tucked under. Repeat on the other side. ○

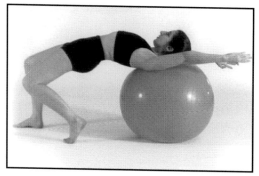

Leg Lifts: Begin in the Basic Flat Back position with your arms out to the side. Lift one leg off the floor and try to hold your balance. The leg may be bent or straight. Repeat on the other side. ○○
Suggested Repetitions: 2 sets

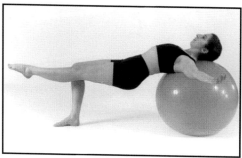

TIPS

✓ As you walk your feet forward, roll through your spine sequentially.

✓ To make it more challenging, hinge from the hip joint, keeping your spine in a solid, neutral position.

✓ For the Leg Lifts, the closer your supporting foot is to the midline of your body, the easier it will be to balance.

MAJOR MUSCLE GROUPS

♦ abdominals
♦ back extensors
♦ gluteals
♦ quadriceps
♦ hamstrings
♦ calves (Heel Raises)

Stretch for: hip flexors

Back Stretch

Basic: Begin sitting on the Ball. Walk your feet forward until your whole back is resting on the Ball. Straighten your legs and reach your arms overhead toward the floor. Just relax into the stretch. ○

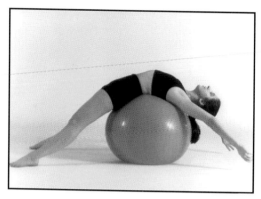

Arm Circles: Begin in the Basic Back Stretch position. Slowly move your arms in as large a circle as possible, letting gravity pull the weight of your arms down toward the floor, increasing the range of motion in your shoulder joints. Reverse the direction. ○
Suggested Repetitions: 3 each direction

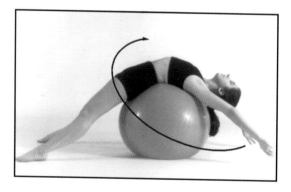
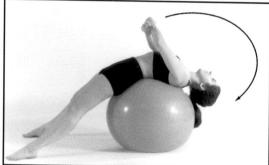

Knee Bends: Begin in the Basic Back Stretch position. Gently bend and straighten your legs, so that your hips flex and move closer to the floor. ⟳
Suggested Repetitions: 8

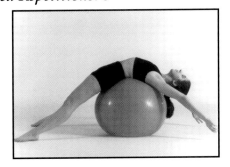 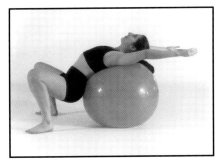

Upper Back Stretch: Begin in the Basic Back Stretch position with your arms out to the side. Roll toward your left side, letting your right knee bend and your right arm circle around overhead to meet the left arm. By reaching both arms toward the left, you should feel a stretch in your upper back. Circle your right arm around overhead to bring you back to the center, then repeat on the other side. ⟳⟳
Suggested Repetitions: 2 sets

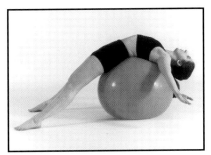 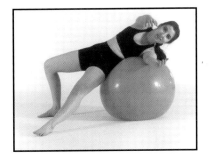

Back Bend Stretch: Begin in the Basic Back Stretch position, but with your feet flat on the floor and your hands on the floor behind you. Gently lift your hips off the Ball so that you are in a back bend. ⟳⟳⟳

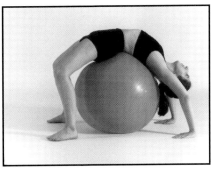

TIPS

✓ When you are ready to sit up, support your neck by placing your hands behind your head, bring your chin to your chest, and walk your feet in as you roll up to a sitting position.

✓ You may keep your hands behind your head to support your neck during the Basic Back Stretch and the Knee Bends.

MAJOR MUSCLE GROUPS

♦ abdominals

♦ quadriceps (Knee Bends)

♦ back extensors (Back Bend Stretch)

Stretch for: back extensors, abdominals, hip flexors, pectoralis, scapular stabilizers (Upper Back Stretch)

Flip-Flop

Begin lying with your mid-back on the Ball and your arms out to the side. Reach your left leg under your right as you roll onto your stomach. From there, continue to roll in the same direction, your right leg reaching under your left, to roll onto your back. Repeat in the other direction. ○○

Suggested Repetitions: 4 each direction

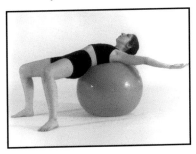 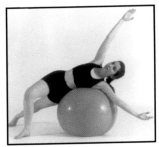

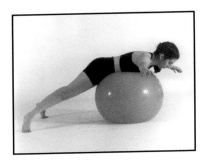 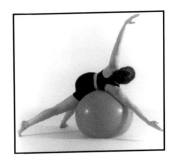

TIPS

✓ Reach your leg out as far as possible, allowing your torso to twist, before you place your foot on the floor.

✓ Be sure that both feet are firmly on the floor before you begin to roll over.

MAJOR MUSCLE GROUPS

♦ abdominals
♦ back extensors

Stretch for: pectoralis, obliques, hip flexors

Leg Press

Lie with your lower back resting comfortably on the Ball and your feet flat against the wall. Keep your spine in a C-curve, and place your hands behind your head to support your neck. Begin with your feet hip-width apart, legs in a parallel position, and knees bent to a 90° angle. From there, straighten and bend your legs. ○

Suggested Repetitions: 10

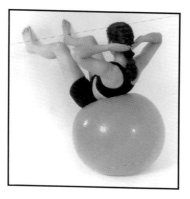

Variation #1: Place your feet apart with your legs turned out. ○

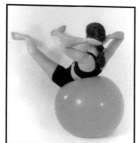

Variation #3: Place your heels together with your legs turned out. ○

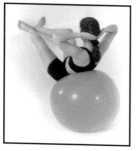

Variation #2: Place your feet together with your legs parallel. ○

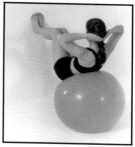

Variation #4: Place your feet together, legs parallel, and on your toes. ○

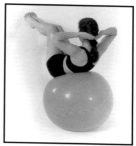

Variation #5: Place your heels together, legs turned out, and on your toes. ◯

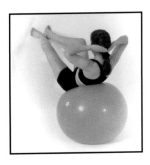

Variation #6: Place only one foot at a time on the wall, keeping your legs parallel. ◯

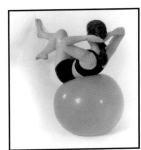

TIPS
✓ Keep equal weight on both feet at all times.
✓ Maintain the C-curve in your spine.

MAJOR MUSCLE GROUPS
- ♦ abdominals
- ♦ quadriceps
- ♦ hamstrings
- ♦ gluteals
- ♦ adductors
- ♦ hip rotators (Variations #1, #3, & #5)

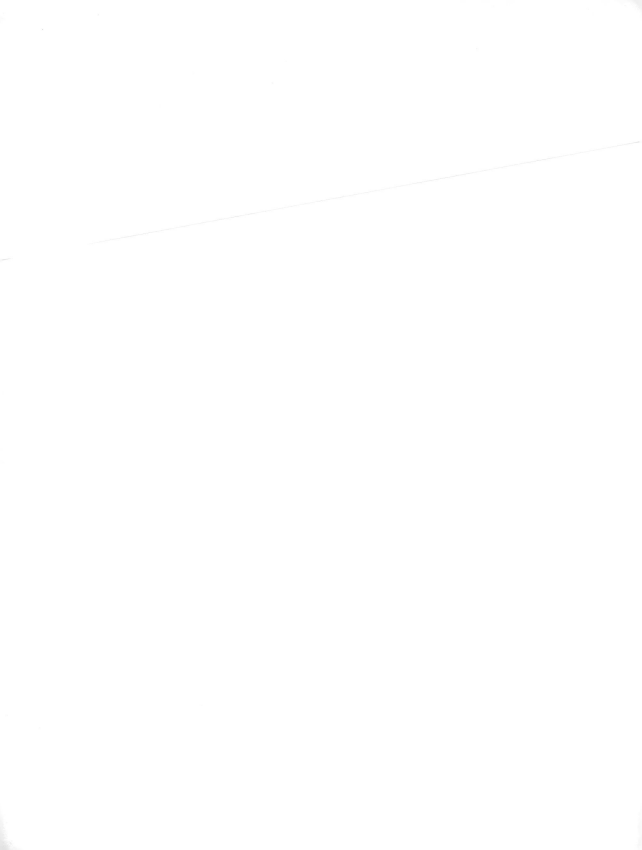

Chapter Four: Lying on the Ball (Prone)

Quadruped

Basic: Lie with your stomach on the Ball and both hands and feet on the floor. Lift your left arm and your right leg off the floor and extend them straight out in a horizontal plane. Try to hold your balance for at least 5 seconds. Repeat on the other side. ○
Suggested Repetitions: 4 sets

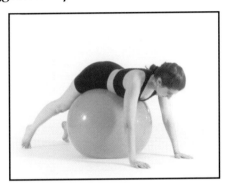 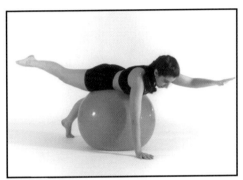

Pulses: Lie with your stomach on the Ball and both hands and feet on the floor. Lift one leg off the floor and extend it straight behind you. Lift and lower your leg in small pulses, moving only a few inches up and down. Repeat on the other side. ○
Suggested Repetitions: 20 each side

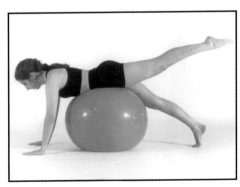

Variation #1: Lift one leg off the floor, your knee bent to a 90° angle and your foot flexed. Pulse your leg up and down as if the sole of your foot is pressing up on the ceiling. ○

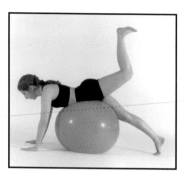

TIPS

✓ Keep your abdominals engaged and your buttocks tight.

✓ Do not lock your elbows.

✓ Do not lift your arm and leg so high that your shoulders or pelvis lose their alignment. Instead, reach out as far as possible in opposite directions, creating a sense of length throughout your body.

✓ When you pulse with a bent leg, keep the shin vertical.

MAJOR MUSCLE GROUPS

♦ back extensors
♦ abdominals
♦ hamstrings
♦ gluteals
♦ scapular stabilizers

Star

Preparation: Lie with your stomach on the Ball and both hands and feet on the floor. Lift your right arm and right leg off the floor and extend them straight out in a horizontal plane. Try to hold your balance for at least 5 seconds. Repeat on the other side. ○

Suggested Repetitions: 4 sets

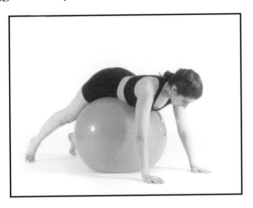 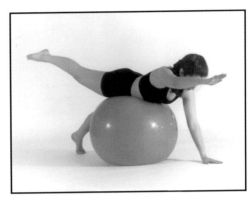

Star: Lie with your stomach on the Ball and both hands and feet on the floor. Lift your left arm and left leg off the floor and up toward the ceiling, rolling on the Ball so that you are facing sideways with only the right side of your body resting on the Ball. From there, lower your arm and leg back down to the floor. Repeat on the other side. ○○○

Suggested Repetitions: 4 sets

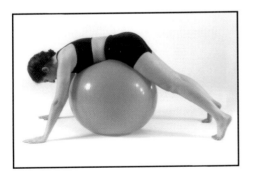 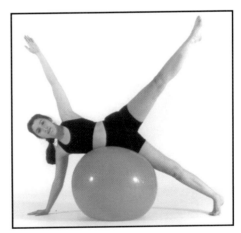

Variation #1: From the Star position, bend your free leg, bringing your toes to the opposite knee. Then straighten your leg back up to the ceiling and complete the exercise. ⚬⚬⚬

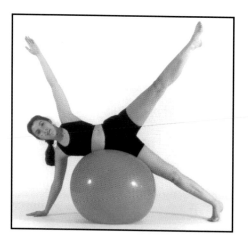 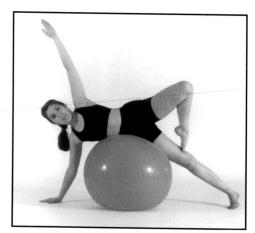

TIPS

✓ Do not lock your elbows.

✓ To make the Star more challenging, lift your arm and leg by reaching them out to your side on the way up to the ceiling, as if you are a door opening on a hinge.

MAJOR MUSCLE GROUPS

- ◆ back extensors
- ◆ abdominals
- ◆ gluteals
- ◆ hamstrings
- ◆ scapular stabilizers
- ◆ hip flexors (Star)
- ◆ abductors (Star)

Stretch for: adductors and hamstrings (Star)

Swan

Lie with your pelvis on the Ball and both feet together on the floor. Placing both hands on the Ball, straighten your arms and lift your chest up into an arch. Then bend your elbows and lower your torso back over the Ball. ◗◯

Suggested Repetitions: 5-8

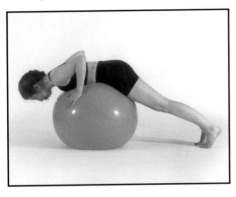 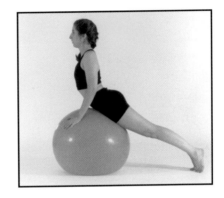

Variation #1: Repeat with one leg turned out and that foot touching the opposite knee. ◗◯◯

Variation #2: Repeat with one leg lifted slightly off the floor. ◗◯◯

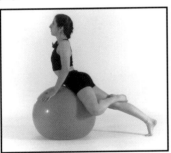 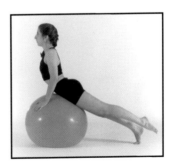

TIPS

✓ Keep your buttocks tight and your pelvis tucked under to protect your lower back.

✓ Engage your shoulder blades as you straighten your arms. Your arms may not straighten all the way. Stay in a range of comfort.

✓ Do not lock your elbows.

MAJOR MUSCLE GROUPS

♦ back extensors
♦ gluteals
♦ abdominals
♦ triceps
♦ scapular stabilizers
♦ hip rotators (Variation #1)
♦ hamstrings (Variation #2)

Stretch for: abdominals, hip flexors, adductors (Variation #1)

Frog

Lie with your pelvis on the Ball and both hands on the floor. Bend your legs and turn them out from the hip joint, so that your knees are apart and your heels are together. Your thighs are in a straight line with your torso. From there, squeeze your buttocks and pulse your legs up and down. Keep your shins vertical as if the soles of your feet are pressing up on the ceiling. ○

Suggested Repetitions: 20

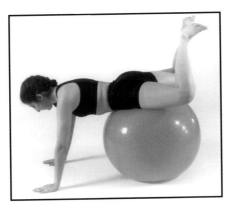

TIPS
✓ Keep your abdominals and buttocks engaged. Do not sink into your lower back.

✓ Do not lock your elbows.

MAJOR MUSCLE GROUPS
♦ back extensors
♦ gluteals
♦ hamstrings
♦ abdominals
♦ scapular stabilizers
♦ hip rotators

Stretch for: hip flexors

Swimming

Lie with your pelvis on the Ball and both hands on the floor. Extend both legs behind you, keeping your body in a long, straight line. From there, flutter your legs up and down in opposition. ○

Suggested Repetitions: 20 sets

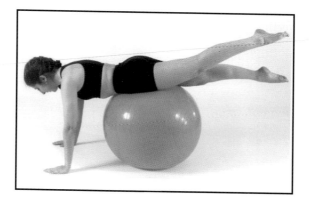

Variation #1: From the Swimming position, click your heels together rapidly. ○

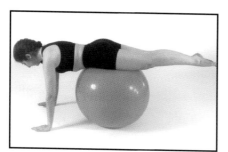

Variation #2: From the Swimming position, cross your legs back and forth at the ankles rapidly. ○

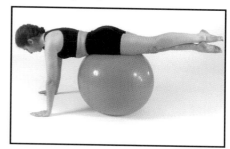

TIPS

✓ Keep your abdominals and buttocks engaged. Do not sink into your lower back.

✓ Keep your legs straight and your feet pointed.

✓ Do not lock your elbows.

MAJOR MUSCLE GROUPS

♦ back extensors
♦ abdominals
♦ hamstrings
♦ gluteals
♦ adductors
♦ scapular stabilizers

One Arm Balance

Lie with your pelvis on the Ball and both hands on the floor. Extend both legs behind you, keeping your body in a long, straight line. From there, lift your left arm off the floor and extend it straight forward. Try to hold your balance for at least 5 seconds. Repeat on the other side. ◯◯

Suggested Repetitions: 4 sets

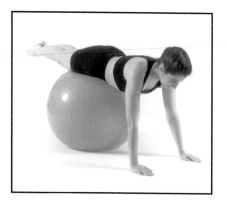 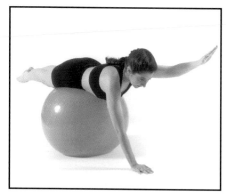

Variation #1: As you lift your arm, also lift the opposite leg. ◯◯◯

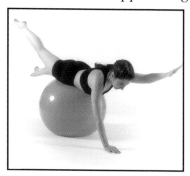

TIPS

✓ Keep your abdominals and buttocks engaged. Do not sink into your lower back.

✓ Keep your inner thighs squeezed together.

✓ Do not lock your elbows.

✓ To increase the difficulty, position the Ball farther away from the center of your body.

MAJOR MUSCLE GROUPS

♦ back extensors
♦ abdominals
♦ hamstrings
♦ gluteals
♦ adductors

Long Stretch

Lie with your pelvis on the Ball and both hands on the floor. Walk your hands forward until your mid-thighs or knees are resting on the Ball. You should be in a long, straight line from head to toe. From there, shift your weight back and forth, moving only at the shoulder joint. ◖○

Suggested Repetitions: 8

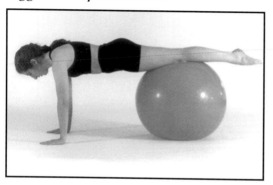 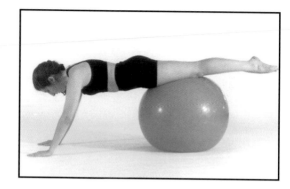

Variation #1: Repeat with one leg lifted off the Ball. ○○○

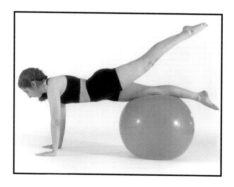

TIPS

✓ Keep your abdominals and buttocks engaged. Do not sink into your lower back.

✓ Keep your inner thighs squeezed together.

✓ Do not let your shoulders move any farther forward than your hands. This is a very small movement.

✓ Do not lock your elbows.

✓ To increase the difficulty, position the Ball farther away from the center of your body.

MAJOR MUSCLE GROUPS

♦ abdominals

♦ back extensors

♦ gluteals

♦ adductors

♦ scapular stabilizers

♦ hamstrings (Variations #1)

Push Ups

Lie with your pelvis on the Ball and both hands on the floor. Walk your hands forward until your mid-thighs or knees are resting on the Ball. You should be in a long, straight line from head to toe. From there, bend and straighten your arms. ◯◯

Suggested Repetitions: 8

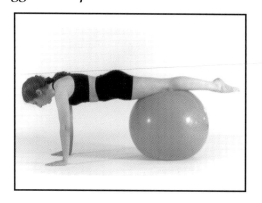 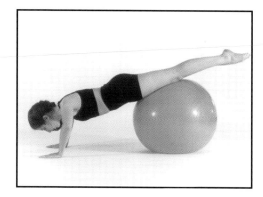

Variation #1: Position the Ball so that your feet are resting on top. ◯◯◯

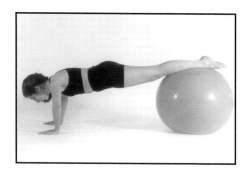

TIPS

✓ Keep your abdominals and buttocks engaged. Do not sink into your lower back.

✓ Keep your inner thighs squeezed together.

✓ Do not lock your elbows.

MAJOR MUSCLE GROUPS

♦ abdominals
♦ back extensors
♦ gluteals
♦ adductors
♦ triceps
♦ pectoralis
♦ scapular stabilizers

Knee Stretch

Basic: Lie with your pelvis on the Ball and both hands on the floor. Walk your hands forward until your mid-thighs or knees are resting on the Ball. You should be in a long, straight line from head to toe. From there, bend your knees in toward your chest, and then press back out to straight legs, rolling the Ball forward and back. When your knees are bent, your shins are resting on the Ball. ⚪⚪
Suggested Repetitions: 8

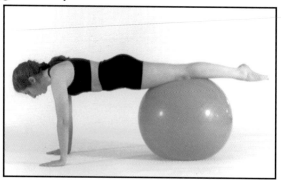 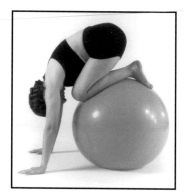

Variation #1: Begin with your ankles on top of the Ball and your knees bent down toward the floor. Roll the Ball backward to straighten your legs, and then bend your knees as the Ball rolls back in. ⚪⚪⚪

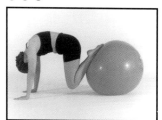 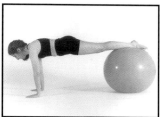

Skier: Repeat the Basic Knee Stretch, but bend your knees in toward one shoulder, rolling the Ball forward on a diagonal. Keep your shoulders still and let your torso twist at the waist. Repeat on the other side. ⚪⚪
Suggested Repetitions: 4 sets

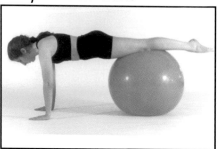 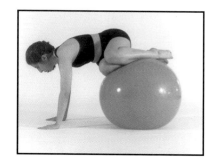

Round Back Stretch: From the Basic Knee Stretch position, move your hands closer to the Ball and round your back all the way over. ○○

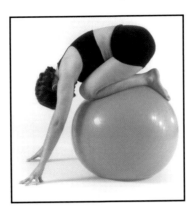

TIPS

✓ Keep your abdominals and buttocks engaged. Do not sink into your lower back.

✓ Keep your inner thighs squeezed together.

✓ Do not lock your elbows.

✓ Round your back as you bend your knees, lifting your stomach up toward the ceiling.

✓ Tuck your head to your chest as you bend your knees in. It will be more difficult to balance when your head is upside-down.

MAJOR MUSCLE GROUPS

♦ abdominals
♦ back extensors
♦ gluteals
♦ adductors
♦ scapular stabilizers
♦ hip flexors
♦ obliques (Skier)

Stretch for: back extensors

Pike

Lie with your pelvis on the Ball and both hands on the floor. Walk your hands forward until your mid-thighs or knees are resting on the Ball. You should be in a long, straight line from head to toe. Keeping your legs straight, bend at the hip joint to lift your hips into a pike position. The Ball rolls in toward you as you fold in half. From there, straighten back out to the starting position. ○○○
Suggested Repetitions: 8

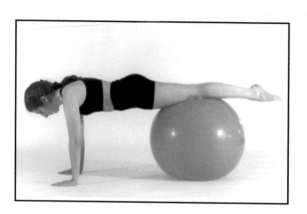 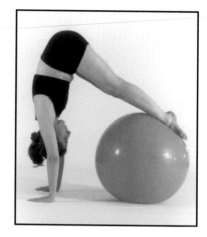

TIPS

✓ Keep your abdominals and buttocks engaged. Do not sink into your lower back.

✓ Keep your inner thighs squeezed together.

✓ Do not lock your elbows.

✓ Tuck your head to your chest as you pike up. It will be more difficult to balance when your head is upside-down.

MAJOR MUSCLE GROUPS

♦ abdominals
♦ back extensors
♦ gluteals
♦ hip flexors
♦ adductors
♦ scapular stabilizers

Scissors

Leg Lifts (Preparation): Lie with your pelvis on the Ball and both hands on the floor. Walk your hands forward until your mid-thighs or knees are resting on the Ball. You should be in a long, straight line from head to toe. Lift one leg off the Ball and try to hold your balance for at least 5 seconds. Repeat on the other side. ○○
Suggested Repetitions: 4 sets

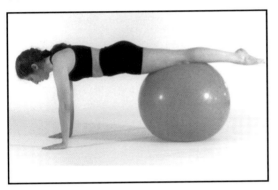
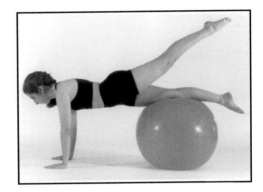

Twist (Preparation): Lie with your pelvis on the Ball and both hands on the floor. Walk your hands forward until your mid-thighs or knees are resting on the Ball. You should be in a long, straight line from head to toe. Twist your body to the left so that your hips are square to the side. Your legs should remain straight. From there, roll back to the starting position. Repeat on the other side. ○○
Suggested Repetitions: 4 sets

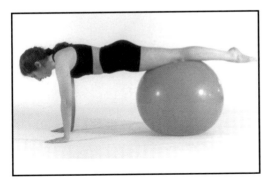
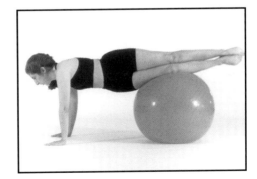

Scissors: Lie with your pelvis on the Ball and both hands on the floor. Walk your hands forward until your mid-thighs or knees are resting on the Ball. You should be in a long, straight line from head to toe. Lift your left leg off the Ball and twist toward the left so that you are resting on the side of your right leg. As you twist, let your legs split apart, reaching your left leg out behind you and your right leg toward the front. From there, bring your legs together as you roll back to the starting position. Repeat on the other side. ○○○

Suggested Repetitions: 4 sets

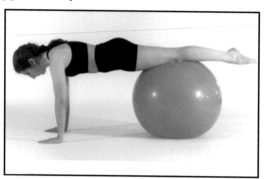 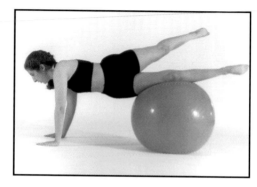

Variation #1: Reach your leg behind you even farther, taking your back into a slight arch. Bend the knee to increase the stretch in your hip flexors, and roll farther away from your hands to get more twist. ○○○

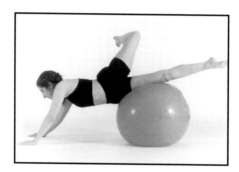

TIPS

✓ Keep your abdominals and buttocks engaged. Do not sink into your lower back.

✓ Do not lock your elbows.

✓ When you arch in Variation #1, be careful not to compress the lower back area.

MAJOR MUSCLE GROUPS

- ♦ abdominals
- ♦ back extensors
- ♦ gluteals
- ♦ scapular stabilizers
- ♦ hamstrings (Leg Lifts and Scissors)
- ♦ adductors (Twist)
- ♦ abductors (Scissors)
- ♦ obliques (Twist and Scissors)

Stretch for: hip flexors and obliques (Scissors)

Diver

Lie with your pelvis on the Ball and both hands on the floor. Extend both legs behind you, keeping your body in a long, straight line. From there, bend your elbows and lift your legs as high as you can. Then straighten your arms and lower your legs back to the starting position. As your legs lift and lower, the Ball may roll back and forth slightly to give momentum. ○○○

Suggested Repetitions: 8

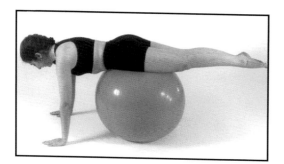

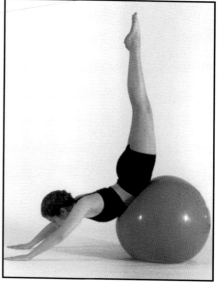

Variation #1: Repeat the exercise with your legs bent and turned out from the hip joint, keeping your knees apart and your heels together (see Frog on page 101). ○○○

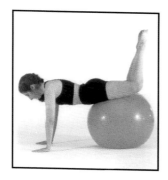
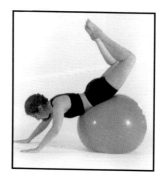

TIPS
✓ Keep your buttocks tight to protect your lower back.

✓ Keep your inner thighs squeezed together.

✓ Do not lock your elbows.

MAJOR MUSCLE GROUPS
♦ back extensors

♦ hamstrings

♦ gluteals

♦ abdominals

♦ adductors

♦ triceps

♦ pectoralis

♦ scapular stabilizers

♦ hip rotators (Variation #1)

Stretch for: abdominals, hip flexors

Flying

Preparation: Lie with your stomach on the Ball and your legs bent. Only your feet should be touching the floor. Press off with your feet and roll forward to catch yourself with your hands. Press back with your arms to land on your feet. ○
Suggested Repetitions: 8

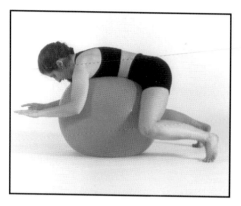 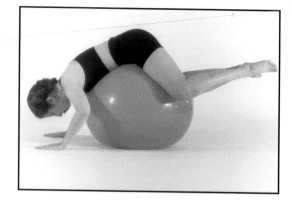

Variation #1: Repeat moving from side to side. ○

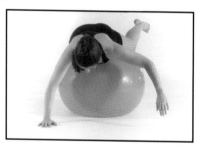

Variation #2: Repeat moving in a circular direction, from your left hand, to your right hand, to your right foot, to your left foot. Reverse the direction. ○

Flying: Repeat the Preparation and try to straighten both arms and legs in the air. There should be a moment immediately after you push off where your arms and legs are all reaching straight out in the air as if you are flying. ◯◯◯
Suggested Repetitions: 8

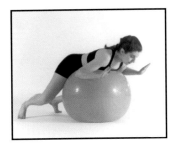 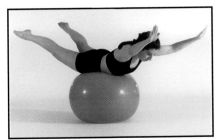 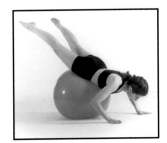

TIPS
✓ Use control so that you land evenly on both hands or both feet.
✓ Do not lock your elbows or your knees when you land. Bend them gently to soften the landing.

MAJOR MUSCLE GROUPS
♦ back extensors
♦ hamstrings
♦ gluteals
♦ quadriceps
♦ triceps
♦ pectoralis
♦ scapular stabilizers
Stretch for: back extensors (Preparation)

Hip Flexor Stretch

Basic: Lie with your stomach and pelvis on the Ball. Place one leg straight behind you and the other bent to the side of the Ball with your foot flat on the floor. Repeat on the other side. ○

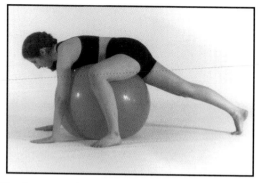

Variation #1: To intensify the stretch, place your hands on the Ball and press up to a more vertical position of the torso. ○○

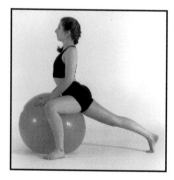

Lunge: From the Long Stretch position (see Long Stretch on page 106), bring one leg forward into a lunge. Keep your back leg straight with either your knee or shin resting on the Ball. Repeat on the other side. ○○○

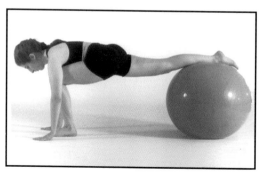

Variation #1: Gently rock back and forth to intensify the stretch. ○○○

TIPS

✓ Keep your buttocks tight and your pelvis tucked under to protect your lower back as you increase the arch in your spine.

✓ Engage your shoulder blades as you straighten your arms. Your arms may not straighten all the way. Stay in a range of comfort.

✓ Do not lock your elbows.

✓ Keep your bent knee over the heel.

✓ For the Lunge, the farther away the Ball is from the center of your body, the more stretch you will feel.

MAJOR MUSCLE GROUPS

♦ abdominals

♦ back extensors (Basic Variation #1)

♦ triceps (Basic Variation #1)

♦ scapular stabilizers (Basic Variation #1)

Stretch for: hip flexors, abdominals (Basic Variation #1)

Round Back Stretch

Lie with your stomach on the Ball, your legs bent, and both hands and feet on the floor. Just let your whole body relax into the stretch. ○

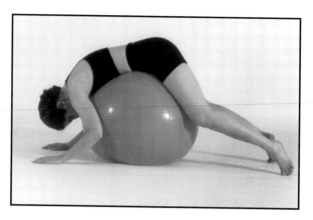

TIPS

✓ Let your head and neck relax completely.

MAJOR MUSCLE GROUPS

Stretch for: back extensors

Adductor Stretch

Lie with your stomach on the Ball and both hands and feet on the floor. Keeping your legs straight, open your legs to the side to stretch your inner thighs. Roll back slightly if needed to intensify the stretch. ○

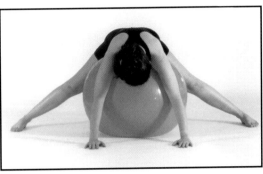

TIPS

✓ You may stretch with the legs in a parallel or turned out position.

✓ Your feet do not need to remain flat on the floor.

MAJOR MUSCLE GROUPS

Stretch for: adductors, back extensors, hamstrings

Pectoralis Stretch

Lie with your stomach on the Ball and both hands and feet on the floor. From there, reach one arm up toward the ceiling, letting your torso twist slightly. Repeat on the other side. ○

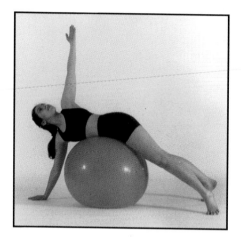

TIPS

✓ Keep your focus on your hand to stretch the muscles in your neck.

MAJOR MUSCLE GROUPS

♦ abdominals

Stretch for: pectoralis, obliques

Quadricep Stretch

Lie with your stomach on the Ball and both hands and feet on the floor. From there, hold onto your left foot with your left hand and pull up slightly toward the ceiling to stretch the front of your thigh. Repeat on the other side. ○○

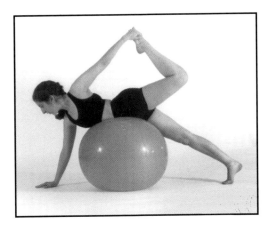

TIPS
✓ Keep your buttocks tight and your pelvis tucked under to protect your lower back.

✓ Do not lock your elbows.

✓ Try to stretch your leg in a parallel position, not off to the side.

MAJOR MUSCLE GROUPS
♦ abdominals

♦ back extensors

♦ scapular stabilizers

♦ gluteals

Stretch for: hip flexors, deltoids

Superman

Lie with your stomach on the Ball and your feet supported against the base of the wall. Keep your legs bent just slightly to avoid locking the knees. With your hands behind your head, raise and lower your torso. ⚬⚬

Suggested Repetitions: **8**

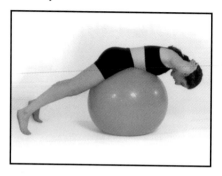 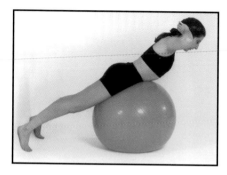

Variation #1: Extend your arms straight overhead. ⚬⚬

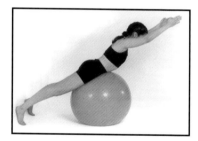

Variation #2: With your arms extended straight overhead, raise your torso up to a vertical position. Then open your arms out to the side, letting your back arch and your knees bend further. Keep your buttocks tight and your pelvis tucked under to protect your lower back. ⚬⚬⚬

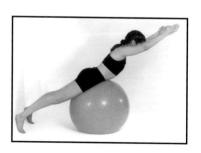 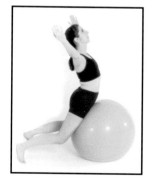

TIPS

✓ Do not hyperextend your spine (except for Variation #2). Raise your torso only until it is in a straight line with your legs, not into an arch.

MAJOR MUSCLE GROUPS

♦ back extensors
♦ hamstrings
♦ gluteals
♦ abdominals

Stretch for: hip flexors, abdominals and pectoralis (Variation #2)

Chapter Five: Lying on the Ball (Sideways)

Side Leg Lifts

Basic: Lie sideways on the Ball with your legs straight and together, so that only your feet and one hand are on the floor. Place your other hand on the Ball to help keep it still. From there, lift and lower your top leg, keeping your legs in a parallel position and your feet flexed. Repeat on the other side. ○○
Suggested Repetitions: 10 each side

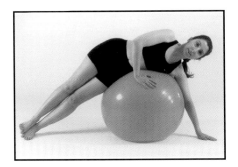 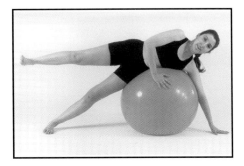

Hip Rotation: Lie sideways on the Ball with your legs straight and together, so that only your feet and one hand are on the floor. Place your other hand on the Ball to help keep it still. Begin by turning your top leg outward, touching your toes to the knee of your bottom leg. Then turn your top leg inward so that both knees touch. Continue alternating between outward and inward rotation. Keep your pelvis completely stable and your working leg bent. Repeat on the other side. ○○
Suggested Repetitions: 8 each side

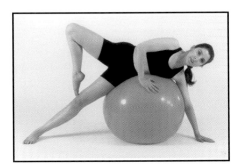 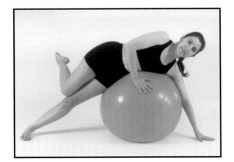

Ballet Extension: Lie sideways on the Ball with your legs straight and together, so that only your feet and one hand are on the floor. Place your other hand on the Ball to help keep it still. From there, touch the toes of your top leg to the knee of your bottom leg. Straighten your leg up toward the ceiling, and then lower it back down to the starting position. Keep your leg turned out from the hip joint the entire time. Repeat on the other side. ○○○

Suggested Repetitions: 8 each side

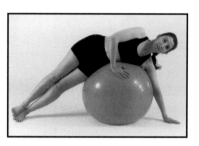 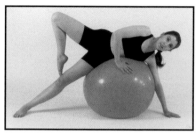 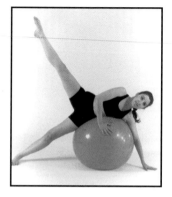

Variation #1: Reverse the movement so that your leg lifts straight up toward the ceiling first. From there, touch your toes to your knee, and then lower back to the starting position. ○○○

Star: Lie sideways on the Ball with your legs straight and together, so that only your feet and one hand are on the floor. Stretch your free arm overhead and lift your top leg off the floor, keeping them both in the same horizontal line. From there, lift your arm and leg up toward the ceiling. Then lower back to the horizontal position. Repeat on the other side. ○○○

Suggested Repetitions: 8 each side

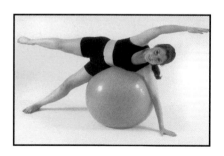 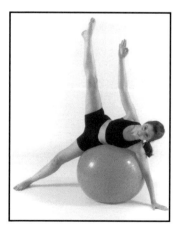

Adductor/Hamstring Stretch: Lie sideways on the Ball with your left hand and foot on the floor. Hold your right foot in your right hand and straighten your leg up toward the ceiling. Repeat on the other side. ○○○

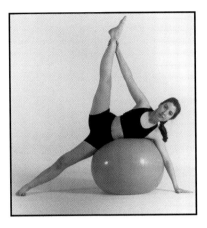

TIPS

✓ Keep your body in a completely straight line from your head to your feet.

✓ Keep your hips square to the front.

✓ Do not lock your elbows.

✓ To increase the difficulty, place your bottom hand on the Ball instead of on the floor.

MAJOR MUSCLE GROUPS

♦ abdominals

♦ back extensors

♦ abductors

♦ gluteals

♦ hip flexors (Ballet Extension and Star)

♦ hip rotators (Hip Rotation, Ballet Extension, and Star)

Stretch for: adductors and hamstrings (Ballet Extension, Star, and Adductor/Hamstring Stretch)

Mermaid

Lie sideways on the Ball with your legs straight and together, so that only your feet are on the floor. Place your bottom hand on the Ball to help keep it still and reach your top arm overhead. Raise your torso up to a vertical position as you reach your top arm out to the side. From there, lower your torso back onto the Ball, raising your arm overhead. Repeat on the other side. ○○○

Suggested Repetitions: 5-8 each side

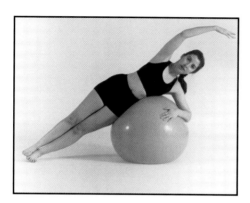 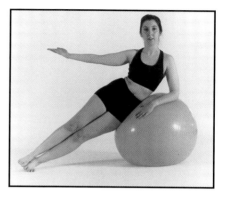

Variation #1: As you raise your torso, also lift your top leg, keeping it in a parallel position. ○○○

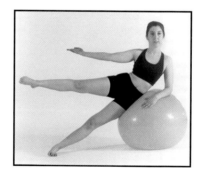

TIPS

✓ Keep your hips square to the front.

✓ Place your feet on the floor slightly apart to help balance, if necessary.

MAJOR MUSCLE GROUPS

♦ abdominals

♦ obliques

♦ back extensors

♦ gluteals

♦ quadratus lumborum

♦ abductors (Variation #1)

Oblique Crunch

Pulses: Lie sideways on the Ball with your top leg crossed in front of your bottom leg. Keep your bottom leg straight and your top leg bent with your foot flat on the floor. From there, twist so that both arms are reaching out toward your legs and pulse your torso up in very small movements. Repeat on the other side. ○○○
Suggested Repetitions: 10 each side

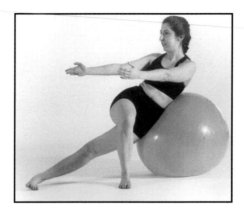

Variation #1: Place your hands behind your head, twist, and lift your torso into a stomach crunch. ○○○

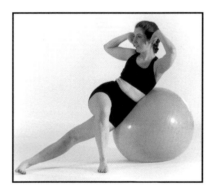

Arm Circles: Lie sideways on the Ball with your top leg crossed in front of your bottom leg. Keep your bottom leg straight and your top leg bent with your foot flat on the floor. Just relax over the Ball and draw very large, slow circles with your top arm. Then reverse the direction of the circle and repeat on the other side. ○

Suggested Repetitions: 3 each direction on each side

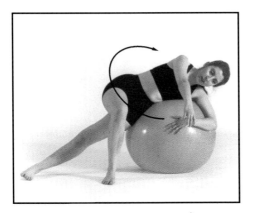 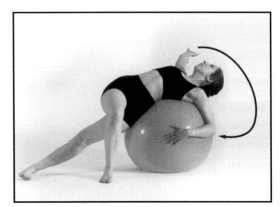

TIPS

✓ Keep your hips square to the front for the Pulses.

✓ You may let your spine twist slightly during the Arm Circles in order to stretch the front of your chest.

MAJOR MUSCLE GROUPS

♦ abdominals

♦ obliques

♦ quadratus lumborum

♦ gluteals

Stretch for: obliques and pectoralis (Arm Circles), gluteals

Side Stretch

Basic: Lie sideways on the Ball with your legs straight, so that only your feet and one hand are on the floor. Place your top leg behind your bottom leg and stretch your free arm overhead. Roll through the Back Stretch position (see Back Stretch on page 86) to the other side and repeat. ○

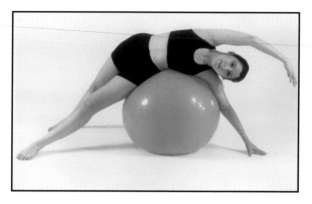

Slide: Begin in the Basic Side Stretch position, with your top leg bent and that foot flat on the floor. From there, slide down toward the floor, bending your top leg even further and opening your top arm to the side. Your bottom leg remains straight as your foot slides along the floor. Then press back to the starting position. Repeat on the other side. ○○

Suggested Repetitions: 4 each side

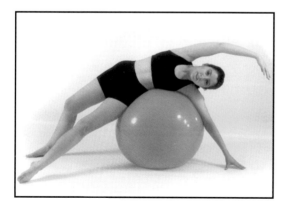
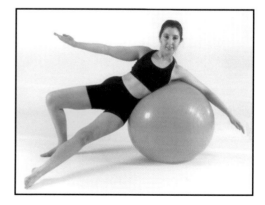

Variation #1: From the Slide position, lift and lower your bottom leg. ◯◯

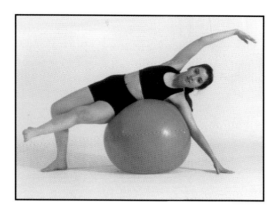

TIPS

✓ The wider your feet, the easier it will be to balance.

✓ To modify the Basic Side Stretch, rest your bottom knee on the floor as you stretch.

✓ For the Slide, be careful not to bend your knee so far that your heel lifts off the floor.

MAJOR MUSCLE GROUPS

♦ abdominals

♦ quadriceps (Slide)

♦ adductors (Variation #1)

Stretch for: obliques

Side Sit Ups

Lie sideways on the Ball with your feet supported against the base of the wall. Only your hip should be resting on the Ball. Keep your bottom leg straight and slightly forward at an angle. Your top leg should be bent and behind your other leg. Keep your knees and inner thighs together. With your hands behind your head, lean out so that you are in a diagonal position from head to feet. From there, raise your torso up to a vertical position, and then lower back to a diagonal. Repeat on the other side. ⭗⭗

Suggested Repetitions: 10 each side

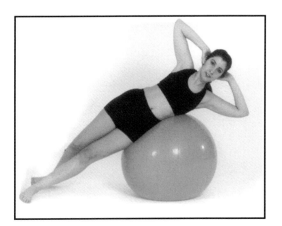 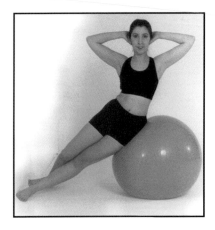

Variation #1: Extend both arms overhead. ⭗⭗

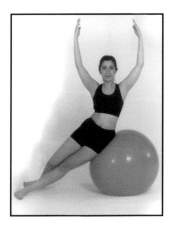

TIPS

✓ Keep your shoulders and hips square to the front.

MAJOR MUSCLE GROUPS

- ♦ abdominals
- ♦ obliques
- ♦ quadratus lumborum
- ♦ back extensors
- ♦ gluteals
- ♦ adductors

Stretch for: obliques

Chapter Six: Standing

Knee Extension

Front: Stand with your left foot on the Ball in front of you, your knee bent to a 90° angle. Keep your supporting leg straight and both legs parallel. From there, straighten and bend your left leg, rolling the Ball back and forth. Repeat on the other side. ○
Suggested Repetitions: 8 each side

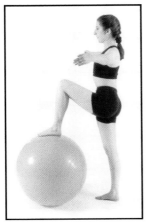 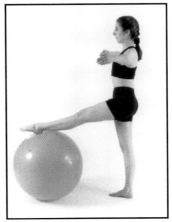

Side: Stand with your right foot on the Ball to your side, your knee bent to a 90° angle. Keep your supporting leg straight and both legs turned out. From there, straighten and bend your right leg, rolling the Ball back and forth. Repeat on the other side. ○
Suggested Repetitions: 8 each side

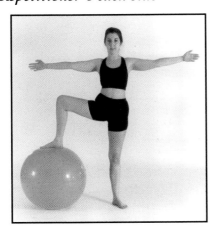 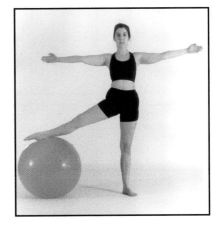

Scooter: Stand with your left shin on the Ball behind you, your knee bent to a 90° angle. Keep your supporting leg slightly bent and both legs parallel. From there, extend and bend your left leg, rolling the Ball back and forth. (Your leg may not straighten all the way.) Keep your pelvis tucked under so that you feel a stretch in your hip flexors. Repeat on the other side. ○

Suggested Repetitions: 8 each side

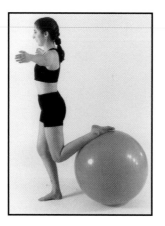 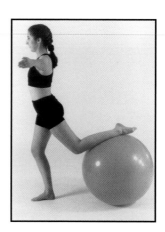

TIPS

✓ As you stand up straight, have good posture in mind, keeping your stomach pulled in, your upper back muscles engaged, and your focus forward.

✓ Try to roll the Ball in a straight line.

✓ Extend your arms out to the side to help balance.

MAJOR MUSCLE GROUPS

♦ abdominals
♦ back extensors
♦ quadriceps
♦ hamstrings
♦ gluteals
♦ hip flexors
♦ hip rotators (Side)

Stretch for: hamstrings (Front), adductors (Side), hip flexors (Scooter)

Hip Rotation

Front: Stand with your right foot on the Ball in front of you, your knee bent to a 90° angle. Keep your supporting leg straight and both legs parallel. From there, rotate your right leg in and out, rolling the Ball from side to side. Repeat on the other side. ◯◯
Suggested Repetitions: 8 each side

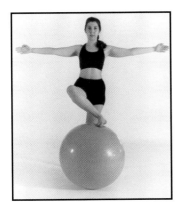 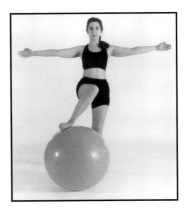

Side: Stand with your left foot on the Ball to your side, your knee bent to a 90° angle. Keep your supporting leg straight and both legs turned out. From there, rotate your left leg in and out, rolling the Ball back and forth. Repeat on the other side. ◯◯
Suggested Repetitions: 8 each side

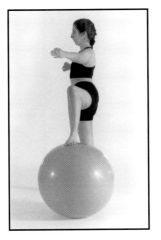 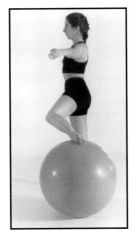

TIPS

✓ As you stand up straight, have good posture in mind, keeping your stomach pulled in, your upper back muscles engaged, and your focus forward.

✓ Keep your working leg bent to a 90° angle and your thigh stationary.

✓ Extend your arms out to the side to help balance.

MAJOR MUSCLE GROUPS

♦ abdominals
♦ back extensors
♦ hip flexors
♦ gluteals
♦ hip rotators

Stretch for: adductors (Side)

Standing Stretches

Front: Stand with your left foot on the Ball in front of you, both legs straight and both arms raised overhead. Bending at the hip joint, reach forward toward your foot so that you feel a stretch in the hamstrings, but do not let your body collapse over the leg. From there, reach your arms out and upward as you bring your torso back to a vertical position. Repeat on the other side. ⭕⭕⭕
Suggested Repetitions: 4 each side

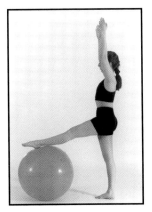 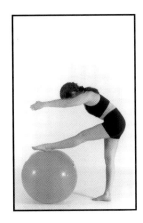

Side: Stand with your right foot on the Ball to your side and both arms raised overhead. Keep both legs straight and turned out. Bending at the waist, tilt toward the Ball so that you feel a stretch in the side of your body, letting your weight lean slightly into your supporting hip. From there, reach your arms out and upward as you bring your torso back to a vertical position. Repeat on the other side. ⭕⭕⭕
Suggested Repetitions: 4 each side

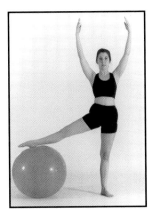 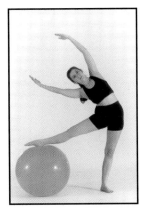

Arch: Stand with your left shin on the Ball behind you, your knee bent to a 90° angle. Keep your supporting leg slightly bent and both legs parallel. Raise both arms overhead and arch your back slightly, taking your focus up toward the ceiling. Then bring your spine back to neutral. Repeat on the other side. ○○○
Suggested Repetitions: 2 each side

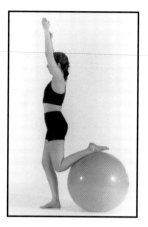 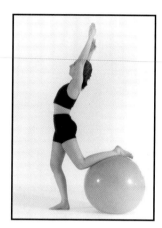

TIPS
- ✓ You may let your leg turn out when you stretch to the front.
- ✓ When you arch to the back, keep your pelvis tucked under to protect your lower back.

MAJOR MUSCLE GROUPS
- ♦ abdominals
- ♦ obliques (Side)
- ♦ back extensors (Arch)

Stretch for: hamstrings and back extensors (Front); obliques, abductors, and adductors (Side); pectoralis, hip flexors and abdominals (Arch)

Squats

Stand and place the Ball between your back and the wall. Keeping your feet hip-width apart, bend your knees and hold for at least 5 seconds. Then straighten your legs. ○○
Suggested Repetitions: 10

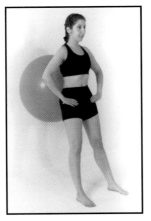 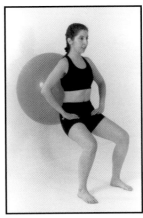

Variation #1: Bend your knees but do not straighten all the way up each time. This can be done in slow pulses. ○○

Variation #2: Keep one leg lifted off the floor, touching that foot to your opposite knee. Both legs are parallel. ○○○

Variation #3: Keep one leg lifted off the floor, extending it straight in front of you. ○○○

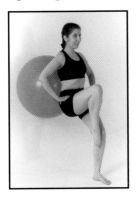 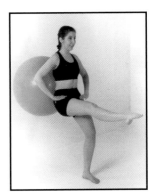

TIPS

✓ When you bend your knees, make sure that your knees are over your heels. If they are over your toes, place your feet farther forward.

✓ Do not bend your knees any farther than 90°.

✓ Work toward holding the position longer and longer each time.

MAJOR MUSCLE GROUPS

♦ quadriceps
♦ abdominals
♦ gluteals
♦ hip flexors (Variations #2 & #3)

Sample Workouts

Advanced ◯◯◯

References

American College of Sports Medicine. *ACSM's Guidelines For Exercise Testing and Prescription.* Pennsylvania: Wilkins & Wilkins, 1995.

Creager, Caroline Corning. *Therapeutic Exercises Using the Swiss Ball.* Colorado: Executive Physical Therapy, 1994.

Friedman, Philip, and Eisen, Gail. *The Pilates Method of Physical and Mental Conditioning.* New York: Warner Books, 1980.

Pilates, Joseph Hubertus, and Miller, William John. *Return to Life Through Contrology.* Nevada: Presentation Dynamics Inc., 1998. (First published in 1945.)

Pilates, Joseph Hubertus. *Your Health.* Nevada: Presentation Dynamics Inc., 1998. (First published in 1934.)

Posner-Mayer, Joanne. *Swiss Ball Applications for Orthopedic & Sports Medicine.* Ball Dynamics International, 1995.

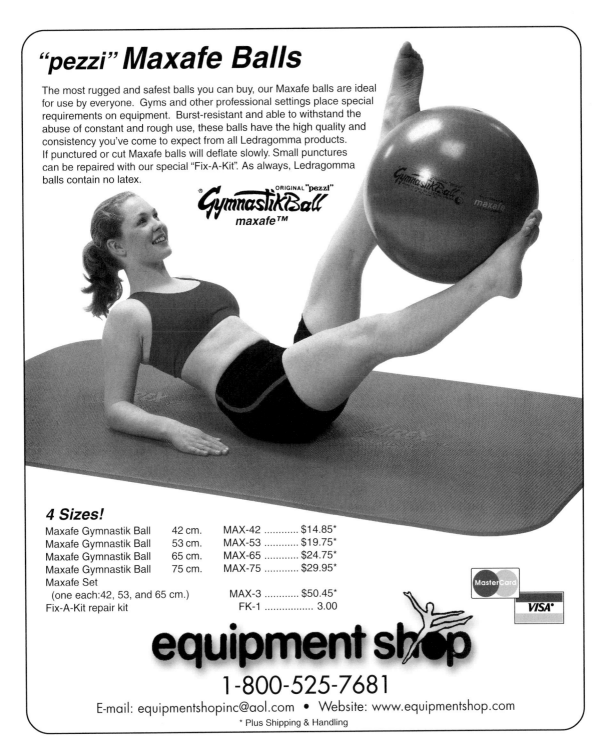